Cultural Psychiatry

Advances in Psychosomatic Medicine

Vol. 33

Series Editor

T.N. Wise Falls Church, Va.

Editors

R. Balon Detroit, Mich.
G.A. Fava Bologna
I. Fukunishi Tokyo
M.B. Rosenthal Cleveland, Ohio

Cultural Psychiatry

Volume Editor

Renato D. Alarcón Rochester, Minn./Lima

5 tables, 2013

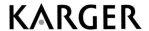

Basel · Freiburg · Paris · London · New York · New Delhi · Bangkok ·
Beijing · Tokyo · Kuala Lumpur · Singapore · Sydney

Advances in Psychosomatic Medicine

Founded 1960 by
F. Deutsch (Cambridge, Mass.)
A. Jores (Hamburg)
B. Stockvis (Leiden)

Continued 1972–1982 by
F. Reichsman (Brooklyn, N.Y.)

Library of Congress Cataloging-in-Publication Data

Cultural psychiatry / volume editor, Renato D. Alarcón.
    p. ; cm. -- (Advances in psychosomatic medicine, ISSN 1662-2855 ; v. 33)
    Includes bibliographical references and indexes.
    ISBN 978-3-318-02394-7 (hard cover : alk. paper) -- ISBN 978-3-318-02395-4
    (e-ISBN)
    I. Alarcón, Renato D. II. Series: Advances in psychosomatic medicine, v.
    33. ; 1662-2855
    [DNLM: 1. Ethnopsychology. W1 AD81 v.33 2013 / GN 270]
    GN270
    155.8'2--dc23
                                                        2013014317

Bibliographic Indices. This publication is listed in bibliographic services, including Current Contents® and Index Medicus.

© Copyright 2013 by S. Karger AG, P.O. Box, CH–4009 Basel (Switzerland) and the American Psychiatric Association (chapter by Drs. R. Lewis-Fernández and N. Krishan Aggarwal)
www.karger.com
Printed in Germany on acid-free and non-aging paper (ISO 9706) by Kraft Druck, Ettlingen
ISSN 0065–3268
e-ISSN 1662–2855
ISBN 978–3–318–02394–7
e-ISBN 978–3–318–02395–4

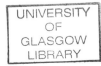

Contents

V

Preface

The fact that a prestigious, specialized book series such as *Advances in Psychosomatic Medicine* decides to publish a volume devoted to cultural psychiatry is eloquent and revealing. The explanation for this is not the celebration of a particular event related to cultural themes, it is not a financially booming enterprise or the promise of commercial success, and it is not an anniversary, not even because of the generous friendship of Tom Wise with this undeserving Guest Editor. To me, the reason is basically an awareness that today, more than at any other point in the history of psychiatry, culture is recognized as truly impregnating every medical or scientific topic, every clinical experience, every diagnosis and every treatment in medicine. Today, more than ever, the perception of wholeness or totality, of integration and honest comprehensiveness in our work as physicians or health professionals, seems to be marking the end of reductionisms of all kinds, and the renewed search for and provision of help to the entire humanity of our patients. That human entity, threatened by bacteria and violence, by viruses and aging, by vascular accidents and by natural disasters, by osteo-muscular and by moral degenerations, by cancers and social stressors, suffers in toto when any of these morbid agents disrupts a sometimes fragile health balance. And culture, being at the primary roots of that humanity, deserves to be managed with the same knowledge and dedication that microorganisms, genes, pathophysiological mechanisms or biochemical formulas receive.

Such being the essential emphasis of this volume, the task of structuring its chapters and finding the right authors with the right credentials was both a pleasurable search and a complex endeavor. The need to present a clear conceptual basis and specific, practical management points dictated part of that search. The principle of balance, invoked above, meant that the chapters should be neither theoretical exercises bordering on academic, preaching-like exhortations nor technical, jargon-charged clichés. Furthermore, the call was for opening the scope, making the issue truly global – culture is, indeed, a global process – and truly international, free of the confessional-like segmentations of schools of thought or national leanings. The roster of authors and the quality of the articles are positive factors in this publication. The mistakes or omissions are the responsibility of the Guest Editor.

After offering a general perspective of the field, an urgent and historically important topic nowadays is, undoubtedly, the connections between culture and psychiatric diagnosis. Two key players in the deliberations on cultural issues related to the development of DSM-5 (Dr. Roberto Lewis-Fernández and Dr. Neil Krishan Aggarwal, both from Columbia University and the New York State Psychiatric Institute) were asked to write the chapter and share their lucid reflections on the topic. The next section expands onto the examination of Cultural Psychiatry realities in the United Kingdom, Sweden, Norway, Germany and France. Dr. Kamaldeep Bhui, Professor of Queen Mary University of London and President of the World Association of Cultural Psychiatry, himself an immigrant, born in Kenya to Indian parents, and educated in the UK, shares his experiences and observations on Cultural Psychiatry in England. Drs. Sofie Bäärnhielm, Cecile Jávo and Mike-Oliver Mösko write objectively about the topic in two Scandinavian countries (Sweden and Norway) and in Germany, considered by many as a geographic key, a political force and a multifaceted door to European culture. They were asked to describe similarities and differences, pluses and minuses of their diverse views on culture and clinical psychiatry. Dr. Joseph Westermeyer, a Professor at the University of Minnesota and distinguished researcher on cultural psychiatry, also presents his unique perspective on the French and Francophile developments in the field.

An important chapter in a volume like this is the one dedicated to transcultural aspects of somatic symptoms, more specifically identified in the context of depressive disorders. Under the direction of Dr. Javier I. Escobar, Associate Dean for Global Health at the University of Medicine and Dentistry of New Jersey, Drs. Issa P. Bagayogo and Alejandro Interian, both also from UMDNJ, coauthor a detailed review of, probably, the most culturally influenced set of symptoms in every region of the world.

The cultural aspects of treatment are presented in the next two chapters. Psychotherapy and its many cultural implications are exemplified by demoralization, a driving force of universal relevance in the help-seeking process of psychotherapy. The chapter is written by Dr. John de Figueiredo from Yale University (himself, a disciple of Jerome D. Frank, the iconic Hopkins researcher who coined and first explored the intricacies of the term) and Sara Gostoli, MA from the University of Bologna, Italy. Ethnopsychopharmacology and pharmacogenomics, two basic sciences with the most extensive scope of clinical research applicability and therapeutic implications are the subject of the chapter written by Dr. Hernán Silva from the University of Chile, a pioneering figure in this field, in Latin America. The goal of these texts was to emphasize more practical implications of the culture-psychiatry interactions.

As it could not be otherwise, the closing chapters deal with research and bioethical considerations in contemporary cultural psychiatry. Research is expectedly complex and truly transcendental, more so in the years and decades ahead. The lead author of the corresponding chapter is Dr. Laurence Kirmayer, Professor of Cultural Psychiatry at McGill University, Chief of the Culture and Mental Health Research Unit of the

Institute of Community and Family Psychiatry in Montreal, Canada, and Editor-in-Chief of *Transcultural Psychiatry*, the most important journal devoted to this field in the world. The bioethical dimensions, substantiating the need for an ethical research approach in psychiatry and cultural psychiatry, are the topic of Dr. Fernando Lolas' chapter; Professor of Psychiatry and Director of the Interdisciplinary Center for Bioethics at the University of Chile, he also served for many years as Director of the Bioethical Division of the Pan American Health Organization (PAHO).

The chapter 'Cultural Psychiatry: A General Perspective' and the 'Epilogue' of this bird's eye view testimony about cultural psychiatry and its contemporary status, both written by the Guest Editor, end with thoughts about the best ways to teach the discipline to practitioners, trainees and even the general public. This is a crucial step if the objective is to maintain the relevance of the discipline and its clinical and academic impact. The volume attempts to be both an updating summary of current achievements in the field, and a call for steady action in its many areas of work now and in the future.

The Guest Editor wishes to express his gratitude to all the distinguished contributors to this volume of *Advances in Psychosomatic Medicine*. Furthermore, it could not have been materialized without the initiative, encouragement and continuous support of Dr. Thomas Wise, Editor-in-Chief of this book series, and the help of the staff at Karger Publishers. We sincerely hope that the genuine interest of our readers will allow them to see the positive features of the issue, and excuse its deficiencies, the exclusive responsibility of its Guest Editor.

Renato D. Alarcón, MD, MPH
Rochester, Minn., USA/Lima, Perú

Alarcón RD (ed): Cultural Psychiatry.
Adv Psychosom Med. Basel, Karger, 2013, vol 33, pp 1–14 (DOI: 10.1159/000348722)

Cultural Psychiatry: A General Perspective

Renato D. Alarcón

Mayo Clinic College of Medicine, Rochester, Minn., USA

Abstract

The current scene in the field of cultural psychiatry shows a vigorous growth, multifaceted conceptual and research developments and more relevant clinical presence. After a pertinent definition of the discipline, this chapter examines the contribution of cultural psychiatry to the etiopathogenesis of mental disorders, to the variations of clinical presentations in numerous entities, to psychiatric diagnosis and treatment and to the relatively unexplored rubric of preventive psychiatry. Advanced concepts of neurosciences and technology-based research can find a place in the realm of biocultural correlates. The role of culture in the definition of mental illness, the renewed notions of the old 'culture-bound syndromes', hope, cognition and culture in psychiatric treatments (including the so-called 'cultural therapies'), and resiliency are areas duly examined and discussed. Cultural psychiatry has re-emerged as a reliable body of knowledge aimed at a comprehensive assessment of human beings as patients.

As the field of contemporary psychiatric research seems to be dominated by the advance of neurosciences, an intriguing parallel development is the increasing recognition of the relevance of culture and cultural factors in practically all aspects of our clinical work [1, 2]. Reluctantly for some, more enthusiastically receptive for many others, this phenomenon reflects an early 21st Century vision of integration, an attempt at a balanced, comprehensive assessment of the complex human realities which science, medicine and psychiatry inevitably deal with. Thus, it should not come as a surprise that the field of cultural psychiatry has re-emerged at this point in history as an epistemological platform, a set of perspectives oriented to a desirable totality in any clinical effort. It is not a subspecialty, not an antineurobiological plot, much less a colorful recitation of exoticisms [3] but a vantage point for thorough mastery of conceptual, diagnostic and therapeutic tasks facing illness and disease both as medical entities and existential labyrinths.

The culture-psychiatry dyad keeps essential correlates of its two component entities: culture as a repository of individual and collective expressions of identity, and psychiatry/mental health as the clinical effort to protect and care for both an individual and a collective sense of well-being, order, stability and perdurability [4]. The latter applies to individuals and groups, communities, countries, world regions or the global scene. It represents physical and emotional harmony in the subject but also a cogent sense of being-in-the world, of true interpersonal and social integration, of freedom, self-determination and wholeness. As elaborate as it is, mental health is also a subtly delicate compositum susceptible to weaknesses or misadventures. When they happen, psychiatry, understood as the comprehensive discipline that it should be, becomes a guardian, a defender or a rational source of protection and care, a powerful tool of rescue and redemption [5].

Culture then plays a variety of roles vis-à-vis the evolvement of mental health/general health. It is the main stage of human life in all its expressions, the scenario at times luminous and at times dark of everyday existence. It is also a script endlessly delineating the transactions between human beings and between them and nature. And culture is also the voice, the attitudes and the actions of us all, players in the comedies and dramas of humankind. Its powerful impact is undeniable, yet it tends to be used either as a plain, 'grab-it-all' notion that explains nothing while pretending to understand everything, or it is simply ignored in the wake of partial pseudo-explanations of human behavior, mental processes or clinical realities.

This is an unquestionable truth, worthy of reiteration: the mental health of the whole world population is being impacted by contemporary developments that, in turn, are shaping a new culture and many subcultures – the so-called globalization phenomenon [6, 7]. To be sure, we should not lose sight of the benefits and advantages of some aspects of the process. No one should deny or minimize the realities of a better communication throughout the entire world, the contributions of cogent debates about global cultural and experiential exchanges, the continuous renewal and increased productivity of art, science and technology [8]. The possibility of and the hope for 'a better future for mankind' seem to be closer at hand. In fact, more or less significant recent political changes in several regions of the world have been considered the result of collective actions fostered by the social networks [9].

The brilliance of geniuses side by side with the efficiency of the average worker can result in promises of betterment for individuals, their families and their communities. People learn to respect others and relearn to be proud of their origins; they can call this, a reinvigorated solidarity [10]. Ottone celebrates *mestizaje* as a sort of well-differentiated cosmopolitan spirit [11], opposed to those like Huntington [12] who conceive of civilization as a series of sadly closed entities. Culture may be indeed a protective-therapeutic tool for health and mental health [13].

Definition and Applications of Contemporary Cultural Psychiatry

The most accepted definition of cultural psychiatry considers it as the discipline that deals with the description, assessment and management of all psychiatric conditions to the extent that they reflect and are subjected to the patterning influence of cultural factors and variables as broad as ethnicity, race and identity or as focused as language, religion, gender and sexual orientation, education, traditions and beliefs, sociodemographic status, dietetic modalities or financial philosophies [14].

The field of cultural psychiatry covers a variety of theoretical and practice areas in all kinds of settings. The fact that formal training programs in schools of medicine and postgraduate centers across the world pay uneven attention to these precepts [15] does not take away their relevance and urgency. They can be applied to etiopathogenic concepts, clinical presentations, diagnostic, therapeutic and prognostic issues as well as to the growing field of prevention. Last but not least, culture plays an anchoring role in the current developments on integrated, multidisciplinary care of all kinds of clinical conditions within a new primary care context called by some, 'behavioral medicine' [16].

Culture and the Etiopathogenesis of Mental Illness

The initial statement in this section must be a sort of disavowal. Nobody would ascertain that cultural factors are etiological agents of mental illness, that is, direct or primary causal events of psychiatric symptoms in any given person; strictly speaking, they may be considered pathogenic factors, those that in one way or another may trigger or contribute to the psychopathological entity evolving as a result of complex *etiopathogenic* interactions, the unique clinical expression of the Engelian biopsychosocial conceptualization [17] to which later, comprehensive-seeking contributions added the cultural and spiritual dimensions [18]. An example of this combination is given by the impact of collective events such as war, terrorism, natural disasters, financial collapses, etc. on culturally based perceptions and actual experiences resulting in the ubiquitous entity known as post-traumatic stress disorder, perhaps more a clinical common denominator than a cogent nosological category [19]. The cultural etiopathogenic view assists in understanding why being poor in the US, being a young Mexican immigrant in North America, and being an Iraqi refugee in Jordan have been all correlated with an increased risk of mental disorder; or the finding that unemployment in the developed world raises a man's risk of early death by 78%, and a woman's by 37% [20]. Be that as it may, such external events or intercultural experiences act as triggers or catalyzers on biopsychosocially vulnerable human beings.

These macro-factors of sociocultural origin may be acute, dramatic and unexpected occurrences leading, in cases, to quite severe clinical outcomes; but they could also be chronic, pervasive, iterative hammering events that do their pathogenic job slowly, longitudinally, in a way that gradually erodes every healthy piece of individual or group identity, every ounce of self-esteem or reparative responsiveness. The most relevant examples come from pathetic stories of domestic violence (systematically enhanced by morning, afternoon and evening news media dispatches), or the cruel, systematic (more hurting when subtler) stigmatizing treatment of the mentally ill and their families. Stigma is indeed a 'double hammer', a strong culture-generated reaction added to the traumatizing experience of mental illness itself [21], becoming then an even more corrosive etiopathogenic factor in psychopathology.

Biocultural connections of different kinds are being increasingly identified as etiopathogenic notions in clinical psychiatry. They consist essentially of biological or physiological responses to or correlates of stressful (pathogenic) events in the patient's psycho-sociocultural surroundings (i.e. family losses, victimization of different kinds, panic-ridden experiences, and culturally developed phobias). The biological correlates of well-delineated cultural factors are measured through technology-based instruments, i.e. neuroimaging, neuropsychological/cognitive and laboratory tests. Admittedly, still away from a reliable biomarkers era [22], some examples of the most promising results of this type of research include: (a) results of clinical and experimental studies (embodiment, early mirror neuron functioning imitating and underlying post-traumatic reenactment) [23]; (b) morphological and physiological size-based changes in key regions of the brain (amygdala, nucleus accumbens, prefrontal cortex, limbic system, interhemispheric connectivity) [24, 25]; (c) endocrine dysregulations (steroids, progesterone, estrogens, oxytocin, thyroid-related compounds) with the HPA axis as the most studied physiopathological site [26]; (d) biochemical reconfigurations (serotonin, dopamine and norepinephrine neurotransmitters, GABA or glutamate-related compounds), and (e) pharmacological effects (including neurotrophic impact of psychotropic agents in different CNS areas) [27, 28].

The field of genetics does not escape from the search of contact points with the world outside genes and their DNA/RNA structure, now expanded to nanomolecular biology, metabogenomics and proteomics [29]. Ethnicity-based differences in pharmacogenomic profiles [30], changes in genetic expressiveness as a result of psychotherapy [31] or the study of creativity and psychopathology provide a fascinating sub-field of inquiry about biocultural links. The sociocultural component in these areas is represented by the generic term 'environment', and the contemporary name for this interaction is epigenetics; 'environment' encompasses facts and findings that go from the uterine content to the macrosocial context, and is recognized as a new and substantial component of the life equation [32]. This terminology also accepts 'endophenotype' as both a repository and a source of clinical manifestations of limited but strong genetic predispositions [33], whereas others have suggested the term 'endosociotype' as expressing genetic basis of strictly social functions and behaviors [34].

Culture and Variations of Clinical Presentations

Culture plays a decisive role in different facets of the clinical presentations of psychiatric entities. The concept of pathoplasty, unfairly neglected in current psychopathological language, conveys the rich connections between culture and the expression of psychiatric symptoms, the way they are described, experienced and reported by patients belonging to different cultures [13, 19, 35]. There is evidence that these details reflect well ingrained factors of historical (i.e. cultural) nature, influencing the content of the symptoms, be they paranoid delusions, manic attitudes or hysterical phenomena. In the contemporary scene, clinical occurrences such as the 'copy-cat' behavior, gross imitation of so-called celebrities, or forms of violence engendered by television series or video games provide powerful pathoplastic data [36, 37].

As culturally charged as the patient's story and symptoms are, the cultural endowment of the clinician is also a most relevant factor in their understanding and comprehension. The clinician's cultural perspective carries modes of appreciation sometimes unchanged by his/her training. It has been demonstrated that Anglo-Saxon psychiatrists tend to pay more attention to cognitive disturbances than to more subjective clinical manifestations, unlike Latin-American, Asian-American or African-American clinicians [38]. Judgments about clinical forms of the same entity, prominence of some symptoms vs. others (cognitive vs. affective manifestations in schizophrenia, for example), assessment of personality features, level of severity and other factors are features strongly influenced by the clinician's cultural background.

The so-called culture-bound syndromes (CBSs) offer a distinctive opportunity of exploration of cultural factors in the clinical presentation of a conglomerate of symptoms. A label first coined by Yap in the 1950s [39], these entities have been long considered semi-autonomous, different from well-known nosological categories (those embedded in Western classifications), almost exclusive to the regions of the world where they were described, and all surrounded by colorful etiopathogenic explanations and symbolic therapeutic rituals led by the solemn figures of shamans, *curanderos, hechiceros*, priests or other folk healers [40]. Practically every corner of the non-Western world, and even some within the West's sphere of influence but carriers of very ancient traditions and history, have produced CBSs using, of course, native language labels: *susto, dhat, Amok, ataque, taijin kiofusho, shenjing-suairuo* and many others. At one point, the clinical world's acceptance of these notions was such that entities like anorexia nervosa and borderline personality disorder were considered 'Western CBSs' [41]. Distinguished researchers from different parts of the world have devoted enormous efforts to the description, characterization and follow-up studies of these entities [42, 43].

Until recently, the consensus in this regard was to maintain CBSs as originally described, that is as idiosyncratic conditions totally related to the beliefs and conceptions of the societies and cultures of origin. Yet, in the last decade, the consideration of similarities between CBSs and diagnoses present in existing nomenclatures seems to be leading to their inclusion under those rubrics or as 'variations' of well-established entities (anxiety or panic disorders, obsessive-compulsive or conversion disorders, even psychotic-like manifestations). To be sure, some CBS will stay as such in forthcoming nomenclatures (DSM-5 included) but their number will be reduced and their descriptions more tightly elaborated [44, 45].

Culture and Psychiatric Diagnosis

World psychiatry has been actively involved for the last several years in the complex process of elaboration of new versions of the two main classification systems of mental disorders, the American Psychiatric Association's DSM-5 and the World Health Organization's ICD-11. The efforts by the two organizations, to assure a 'harmonization' of the systems allow the possibility that culture will be given its rightful place in the new nomenclatures.

The DSM-5 has a section on Cultural Aspects of Psychiatric Diagnosis which includes explanations of the main cultural postulates of diagnosis in psychiatry, reviews the history of these efforts in past versions of the system, and outlines the main new proposals. It does not include, however, something that many consider essential in any attempt to solidify the role of culture in psychiatry in general: whether there is a cultural component in the basic definition of mental illness [46], beyond the standard disclaimer that mental illness and its manifestations 'do not follow or conform to the requirements of the patient's culture of origin'.

Another aspect of these deliberations is related to the 'nosological location' of the Cultural Syndromes, mentioned above. There is also a section of cultural/clinical concepts, replacing the Glossary in DSM-IV's Appendix I [47]. The elaboration of the Cultural Formulation Interview (CFI), an instrument purporting to provide a more precise, fluid and graphic detail of the different sections of DSM-IV TR Appendix I's Cultural Formulation (CF) [48], and discussed in the chapter by Lewis-Fernández and Aggarwal [this vol.], is the most significant addition to the cultural content of DSM-5. Finally, cultural undercurrents, born in the social macro-context and processed through patient, family and clinician interactions, generate a dynamics of unique characteristics [49]. Jerome Frank's classical work [50] describes the patient's 'assumptive world' as a crucial component of the encounter, a concept obviously loaded by cultural material. The clinician must pay attention to issues of meaning and context, either to certify pathology or de-pathologize behaviors known and accepted by the patient's culture [13]; he/she must also inquire about the patient's help-seeking journeys, and collect the patient's explanations about eventual culture-inspired causes of his or her emotional ailments. Needless to say, as Kleinman and Kleinman [51] demonstrated in their research on 'neurasthenia' in China, sometimes surprising diagnostic realities may emerge.

Culture and Psychiatric Treatment

From a general perspective, we certainly don't want to fall into the 'cultural trap' outlined in 1930 by no other than Pierre Janet [52]: 'If a patient is poor, he is committed to a public hospital as 'psychotic'; if he can afford the luxury of a private sanitarium, he is put there with the diagnosis of 'neurasthenia'; if he is wealthy enough to be isolated in his own home under constant watch of nurses and physicians, he is simply an indisposed 'eccentric'.' Carrying a massive cultural message, this statement certainly sounds very contemporary.

It is clear that in each of the two main treatment approaches to mental illness (pharmacotherapy and psychotherapy), culture has introduced elements of undeniable relevance. The history of psychiatry tells us that 'in the beginning', the management of emotional or behavioral symptoms was essentially psychotherapeutic via rituals and prayers, invocations or lyrics. Both faith and suggestibility were used in efforts to favor a return to the normality of the times and the society at large [53, 54]. Culturally strong sources such as religion or ethics provided tools that gradually accentuated issues of hierarchy and authority, knowledge and social sanction of the actions and procedures of healers of different persuasions but with common objectives: to treat the deviant, the sinner, the bewitched or the *loco* [55]. History lent a hand to make psychoanalysis the liberating incarnation of anti-Victorian rebellions or revenges [56, 57].

Current fashionable procedures such as CBT or DBT use, in spite of their cognitive base, beliefs and behaviors strongly supported by cultural referents, including yoga, *tai chi* or other relaxation exercises [58]. The multiplication of psychotherapeutic schools in the last 100 years also testifies to the same, very human search for answers to enigmatic or mysterious ailments. Even the use of technical jargons or especially designed terms (transference, exorcism, mentalization, *dasein*) quite probably reflect also the human tendency to use the 'uniqueness' of new dressings in contemporary versions of old truths.

The therapeutic value of almost exclusively cultural factors such as religion and spirituality has been confirmed time and time again [54]. The 'cultural dynamics' of the psychotherapeutic encounter plays a relevant role in this process [49]. Inspired by Frank's fascinating articulation of the 'common ingredients of all psychotherapies' [49, 59], the mixing of patient and clinician's perspectives, when symmetric and harmonious, becomes the most powerful therapeutic element of them all. Actually, the concept of 'common ingredients' is the strongest vindication of culture as a therapeutic element: hope, trust, faith, respect, institutional support sanctioning credibility as guarantee of knowledge and competence are all factors shaped by the surrounding culture. Demoralization is also the universal, ultimate reason for the patient to seek help. The patient goes to see the therapist because society tells him/her so, and society extracts its advice from the conviction of culturally based processes: training, transmission of knowledge and expertise, pursuit of wisdom and excellence [60].

The processes go on. The growth of so-called minority populations in many present-day societies and the unique characteristics of emotional suffering among some of their members, has led to the elaboration of many 'cultural psychotherapies'. Names such as Morita therapy, *Dichos* therapy, *Tai chi*, and others [61, 62] represent particular efforts by mental health professionals to provide counsel and support to patients using their own resources: language and interaction styles, but most importantly concepts dear to the patient's cultural, family or social environment, procedures they feel comfortable with, even theoretical principles attuned to their subjective needs and expectations. Several comparative research studies of cultural and conventional psychotherapies in selected patient samples have proven the correctness of these approaches [63].

Half way between psychotherapy and pharmacotherapy, history recognizes the therapeutic use of hallucinogens or psychedelic agents [64] as a controversial chapter that, nevertheless, seems to be looking for another clinical and heuristic opportunity. Based on traditional habits and word-of-mouth through generations, the use of peyote and other mushrooms, psylocibin, cocaine or *ayahuasca* had a strong cultural basis and even clinical confirmation of effectiveness (particularly in cases of alcoholism and substance abuse during the 1950s and early 1960s) before their arrival to university campuses and cult-inspired abuse with stories of habituation, irreversible sequelae, physical ailments and subsequent criminalization shut them out of established research settings and destroyed academic careers in the process [65]. Several authors in recent years and in different parts of the world seem to be determined to renew efforts to seriously study these possible therapeutic applications [66, 67].

The practice of pharmacotherapy has, unwittingly, become a sort of 'subculture' by delineating a substantial part of the identity of today's psychiatrist, that is, the 'biological' or 'scientific' approach to treatment as described by its defenders, or the 'pill dispenser' characterization in the eyes of its detractors, far away from the comprehensiveness embodied by the joint application of psychotherapy. It is a well-known fact that many psychiatrists now throughout the world (but, admittedly, more so in developed continents) circumscribe their practice to a more or less superficial diagnostic assessment followed by the relatively quick decision to prescribe medications. The choice of the pharmacological agent may be based on literature reports but, perhaps in most cases hardly follows scientific reasons: 'experience', cost, intuition, recent marketing arrival or, perhaps, sharing of a good response to the same medication by a family member with a similar clinical presentation. The underlying force, according to many critics of this trend, is the influence (subtle or stentorian, deliberately commercial or academically customized) of the pharmaceutical industry's systematic advertisement [68]. Two recent articles by Marcia Angell, former Editor of the *New England Journal of Medicine* published in a prestigious literary magazine [69, 70], as reviews of several books on the subject [71–73] led not only to a vigorous response by the then President of the American Psychiatric Association [74] but also to a renewed debate about the topic. Culture disrupting psychiatry or, as others put it, the 'culture of psychiatry' being perturbed at its roots by forces beyond its control.

A much more transparent example of connections between psychopharmacotherapy and culture is the entry of pharmacogenomics in the clinical stage [30, 75], during the last decade and a half, as discussed in the chapter by Silva [this vol.]. Pharmacogenomics is linked to culture through the cultural entity called ethnicity [76]. There is evidence of differences in the genotypic profile of ethnic groups when tested for delineation of their metabolic capabilities with psychotropic agents. Thus, the clinician will not have to use the same doses for all patients, as a closer attention will have to be paid to the patient's background and physiognomy, until recently a simple formalistic procedure. Further research at both basic and clinical levels will throw more light onto this innovative modality of treatment. Mrazek and Lerman's [77] proposal of conducting pragmatic clinical trials instead of randomized ones has already attracted due attention.

In the field of treatment, another change in practice dictated by cultural realities has to do with the demographics of the workforce: the number of psychiatrists and even of all mental health professionals across the world is insufficient to provide adequate care to increasing volumes of patients [78]. Another consequence of the massive social changes enumerated above, this reality, plus other logistic considerations in modern approaches to patient care, is leading to probably one of the most constructive and creative strategies evolving nowadays: an integrative and more focused training of and support to Primary Care specialists and nonmedical professionals (nurses, physician assistants, social workers) in traditional and nontraditional settings (including rural and deprived areas) [16, 79]. If the practice of telepsychiatry as part of telemedicine also expands as its advocates hope and some have already demonstrated [80, 81], the world will witness another great example of contemporary cultural realities (this in the form of electronic technology) contributing to effective and efficient psychiatric care.

Culture and Prevention in Mental Health

In the mental health field, an adequate understanding of all cultural variables and of their mutual interactions, as well as an accurate measurement of severity levels in impending or declared psychopathologies would be a first step on the road to prevention. Systematic and massive efforts in public and professional education can consolidate initiatives of many kinds in well-conceived public health campaigns adapted to the cultural milieu of the target populations. Multidisciplinary teams should be the main tool to be structured and used in an atmosphere of genuine respect for everybody's contributions – another necessary cultural change in an era in which, at different levels but in all parts of the world, the hierarchization of different mental health professions continues to be a pervasive cultural malady.

One topic that has attracted growing attention from scientists and administrators, academicians, bureaucrats and even politicians, is resiliency. Initially depicted more as a literary metaphor (even though its etymological origin resides in the science of physics – from the Latin word *Resilire* or 'leap back', the capacity of an object to return to its original form after being bent, compressed or stretched out of shape), it gradually became the matter of philosophical reflections as well as historical accounts, ethnic and sociocultural comparisons, biological research as well as media interest [82, 83]. Inevitably, it entered the health and clinical realms with the obvious but, until relatively recently, neglected implication of being a protective factor against adversities of all kinds: physical health problems, psychological injuries and declared psychopathologies. The conclusion was that, in such context, the volume and reinforcement of resiliency would be valuable tools in preventive efforts. Pronouncements by prestigious organizations like the Institute of Medicine in the US [84] and increasing research in both neurobiological [85] and psychosocial [86] areas has made of this precious cultural concept a point of convergence articulating the characteristics of a 'resilient personality' [87], and the notion that fostering resiliency along the developmental cycle would probably be an extraordinary contribution to prevention in the mental health field.

Discussion

A summa summarum of the impact of culture on diagnostic, treatment and prevention efforts in the psychiatric field (as part of the medical scope) is the continuous improvement and, more so, the optimization of what has been called quality of life, the matter of specific measurement instruments in clinical psychology, psychiatry and psychotherapy [88, 89]. It becomes the ultimate cultural goal for individuals and societies alike; it is proclaimed by political leaders, social scientists, philosophers, historians and the average citizen as a worthy existential objective beyond materialistic, demagogic or overidealized life scripts [90, 91]. It has to do with the need for a rational and fair coverage of mental health problems, and an adequate distribution of public and private financial resources. It goes beyond the boundaries of doctrinary or ideological camps to embrace a truly human, universal aspiration. In the best ethical perspective, a good quality of life embodies integrity, altruism, freedom and solidarity. Some call it a full sense of self-realization [92].

Thus, the relevance of culture and cultural factors in today mental health across the globe has gained strength in recent decades. It has not been an easy journey given the complexities and risks of such an enterprise, the current scope and understanding of the field, and the specific connections of culture with different aspects of psychiatric work [44, 45, 75, 93]. The study of conceptual and factual dilemmas of contemporary psychiatry, such as the homogeneity/heterogeneity conundrum [18, 94] determined by different historical, social, political and cultural events in the contemporary world scene, somehow leads also to the exploration of such connections.

Cultural factors in the etiopathogenesis of mental conditions, from a macro- to a micro-factorial causality, and in the various forms of clinical presentations and the varying perspectives of patient, clinician, relatives and others, ought to be studied. Similarly, cultural psychiatry has made substantial contributions to the field of diagnosis, to be tested in the developmental processes of the new nomenclature systems in world psychiatry; issues such as cultural identity, causal attributions, and cultural syndromes are some of the issues to be evaluated through the new Cultural Formulation Interview [14, 41, 48, 95, 96]. Culture and psychiatric treatment have their own dynamic interactions and involve the development of specific cultural techniques as well as the growth of scientific practices such as pharmacogenomics and its ethnic variations. In mental health prevention, culture provides a truly multidisciplinary perspective, fosters the study and use of resiliency and contributes decisively to the shaping of a positive quality of life [87, 97].

Conclusions

Cultural factors are the focus of growing studies in the conceptual, clinical and research-oriented aspects of medicine and psychiatry. In fact, cultural psychiatry has re-emerged as a reliable body of knowledge aimed at a comprehensive consideration, assessment and management of all kinds of clinical entities. The connection of cultural determinants in the etio-pathogenesis of mental conditions, their diagnosis, treatment, outcome and prognosis broadens the perspectives of every clinician. Particular attention is being paid to the recognition of culturally based modalities of help-seeking, explanatory models of illness and idiosyncratic patterns of management, including the fostering of resiliency. The impact of cultural factors on physical health and as a factor in the subsequent deployment and use of multidisciplinary approaches to primary medical care are urgent topics of study [16, 78, 98]. Progress has been made thanks to the work of pioneers in the past, and their historical heirs, seasoned leaders of the present in different parts of the globe. This entails a promise of more research at basic and translational levels, better didactics and improved resources for a more solid practice in the future.

References

1 Kohn R, Wintrob RM, Alarcón RD: Transcultural psychiatry; in Sadock BJ, Sadock AE, Ruiz P (eds): Comprehensive Textbook of Psychiatry, ed 9. Philadephia, Lippincott Williams & Wilkins, 2009, vol 1, pp 734–753.

2 Tseng WS: Handbook of Clinical Psychiatry. San Diego, Academic Press, 2001.

3 Alarcón RD: What cultural psychiatry isn't. Psychline 1998;2:27–28.

4 World Health Organization: The World Health Report. Mental Health: New Understanding, New Hope. Geneva, World health Organization, 2001.

5 Frank JD: Psychiatry, the healthy invalid. Am J Psychiatr 1977:134:1340–1355.

6 Stiglitz J: Globalization and Its Discontents. London, Penguin Books, 2002.

7 Atasoy Y: Explaining globalization; in Atasoy Y, Carroll V (eds): Global Shaping and Its Alternatives. Bloomfield, Kumarian Press, 2003, pp 3–12.

8 Chorost M: World Wide Mind: The Coming Integration of Humanity, Machines and the Internet. New York, Free Press, 2011.

9 Halpern S: The iPad Revolution. New York, Rev Books, 2010, pp 23–26.

10 McNeely IF, Wolverton L: Reinventing Knowledge: From Alexandria to the Internet. New York, Norton, 2010.

11 Soto H: La globalización y su domador. Entrevista con Ernesto Ottone. La Tercera (Santiago de Chile), 8 de Mayo, 2011, pp R21–R23.

12 Huntington SP: The Clash of Civilizations and the Remaking of World Order. New York, Simon & Schuster, 1996.

13 Alarcón RD, Foulks EF, Westermeyer J, Ruiz P: Clinical relevance of contemporary cultural psychiatry. J Nerv Ment Dis 1999;187:465–471.

14 Group for the Advancement of Psychiatry, Committee on Cultural Psychiatry: Cultural Assessment in Clinical Psychiatry. Washington, American Psychiatric Publishing, 2002.

15 World Psychiatric Association Education Committee: Report on Psychiatric Education Programs across the World. Presented at the World Congress of Psychiatry, Buenos Aires, 2011.

16 Feldman MD, Berkowitz SA: Role of Behavioral Medicine in Primary Care. Curr Opin Psychiatry 2012;25:121–127.

17 Engel GL: The clinical application of the biopsychosocial model. Am J Psychiatr 1980;137:535–543.

18 Ghaemi S: The Concepts of Psychiatry: A Pluralistic Approach to the Mind of Mental Illness. Baltimore, Johns Hopkins University Press, 2003.

19 Kleber RJ, Figley CR, Gersons BPR (eds): Beyond Trauma. Cultural and Societal Dynamics. New York, Plenum Press, 1995.

20 Kunzig R: Seven Billion. National Geographic Magazine, 2011, pp 42–69.

21 Stuart H: Lucha contra la estigmatización causada por trastornos mentales: perspectivas pasadas, actividades presentes y direcciones futuras. World Psychiatry (Spanish Ed) 2008;6:185–188.

22 Hyman SE: The diagnosis of mental disorders: the problem of reification. Ann Rev Clin Psychol 2010;6:155–179.

23 Gaensbauer TJ: Embodied simulation, mirror neurons, and the reenactment of trauma in early childhood. Neuropsychoanalysis 2011;13:81–97.

24 Ochsner KN, Knierim K, Ludlow DH, Hanelin J, Ramachandran T, Glover G, Mackey SC: Reflecting upon feelings: an fMRI study of neural systems supporting the attribution of emotion to self and other. J Cogn Neurosci 2004;16:1746–1772.

25 Singer T, Lamm C: The social neuroscience of empathy. Ann NY Acad Sci 2009;1156:81–96.

26 Prince M, Glozier N, Sousa R, Dewey M: Measuring disability across physical, mental and cognitive disorders; in Regier DA, Narrow WE, Kuhl EA, Kupfer DJ (eds): The Conceptual Evolution of DSM-5. Washington, American Psychiatric Publishing, 2011, pp 189–227.

27 Li X, Frye MA, Shelton RC: Review of pharmacological treatment in mood disorders and future directions for drug development. Neuropsychopharmacology 2012;37:77–101

28 Hoppenbrouwers SS, Farzan F, Barr MS, Voineskos AN, Schutter DJLG, Fitzgeral PB, Daskalakis ZJ: Personality goes a long way: an interhemispheric connectivity study. Front Neuropsycht Imag Stim 2010;1:140–147.

29 Vikas D, Mukta G, Tracy A, Zheo FF: New frontiers in proteomics research: a perspective. Int J Pharmaceut 2005;299:1–18.

30 Mrazek DA: Psychiatric Pharmacogenomics. New York, Oxford University Press, 2010.

31 Kandel ER: Psychiatry, Psychoanalysis and the New Biology of Mind. Washington, American Psychiatric Publishing, 2005.

32 Klass P: 'Environment' Poses a Knotty Challenge in Autism. The New York Times, August 9, 2011, p D5.

33 Flint J, Munafo MR: The endophenotype concept in psychiatric genetics. Psychol Med 2007;37:163–180.

34 Alarcón RD: Psychiatric Pharmacogenomics: Research delineations and clinical perspectives. 11th Spanish Congress of Psychiatry, Santiago de Compostela, 2007.

35 Kennedy DP, Adolphs R: Social neuroscience: stress and the city. Nature 2011;474:452–472.

36 Lynch E: La vida en serie. El Pais (Madrid, Spain), Setiembre 27, 2011, p 29.

37 Beck AT, Brown G, Steer RA, Eidelson JI, Riskind JH: Differentiating anxiety and depression: a test of the cognitive content-specificity hypothesis. J Abnorm Psychol 1987;96:179–183.

38 Turkle S: Alone Together: Why We Expect More from Technology and Less from Each Other. New York, Basic Books, 2011, p 154.

39 Yap PM: Mental diseases peculiar to certain cultures: a survey of comparative psychiatry. J Ment Sci 1951;97:313–327.

40 Castillo RJ: Lessons from folk healings; in Tseng WS, Streltzer J (eds): Culture and Psychotherapy. A Guide to Clinical Practice. Washington, American Psychiatric Press, 2003, pp 81–101.

41 Lester RJ: The (dis)embodied self in anorexia nervosa. Soc Sci Med 1997;44:479–489.

42 Villaseñor SJ: Apuntes para una Etnopsiquiatría Mexicana. Guadalajara, Imprenta Universitaria, 2008.

43 Guarnaccia PJ, Lewis-Fernández R, Martínez Pincay I, Shrout P, Guo J, Torres M, Canino G, Alegría M: *Ataque de nervios* as a marker of social and psychiatric vulnerability: results from the NLAAS. Int J Soc Psychiatry 2010;56:298–309.

44 Alarcón RD: Culture, cultural factors and psychiatric diagnosis: review and projections. World Psychiat 2009;8:1–9.

45 Kirmayer LJ, Minas H: The future of cultural psychiatry: an international perspective. Can J Psychiatry 2000;45:438–446.

46 Bolton D: What Is Mental Disorder? An Essay in Philosophy, Science and Values. Oxford, Oxford University Press, 2008.

47 American Psychiatric Association: Diagnostic and Statistical Manual for Mental Disorders, ed 4. (DSM-IV) Appendix I (Outline for Cultural Formulation and Glossary of Culture-Bound Syndromes). Washington, APA, 1994, pp 843–849.

48 Lewis-Fernandez R: The cultural formulation. Transcultural Psychiatry 2009;46:379–382.

49 Alarcón RD, Frank JB, Williams M: Cultural dynamics in psychotherapy and cultural psychotherapies; in Alarcón RD, Frank JB (eds): The Psychotherapy of Hope. The Legacy of Persuasion and Healing. Baltimore, Johns Hopkins University Press, 2012, pp 281–309.

50 Frank JD: Persuasion and Healing. A Comparative Study of Psychotherapy, ed 2. Baltimore, Johns Hopkins University Press, 1973.

51 Kleinman A, Kleinman J: Somatization: The interconnections in Chinese society among culture, depressive experiences, and the meanings of pain; in Kleinman A, Good B (eds): Culture and Depression. Studies in the Anthropology and Cross-Cultural Psychiatry of Affect and Disorder. Berkeley, University of California Press, 1985.

52 Janet PM: Quoted in Lapham's Quarterly 2009;2:53.

53 Thubron C: The Last Shaman. New York, Rev Books, 2011, pp 56–57.

54 Griffith JL: Psychotherapy, religion and spirituality; in Alarcon RD, Frank JB (eds): The Psychotherapy of Hope. Baltimore, Johns Hopkins University Press, 2012, pp 310–325.

55 Micale MS, Porter R (eds): Discovering the History of Psychiatry. New York, Oxford University Press, 1994.

56 Roazen P: Freud and His Followers, ed 4. New York, New York University Press, 1984.

57 Robert M: The Psychoanalytic Revolution. Sigmund Freud's Life and Achievement. New York, Avon Books, 1966.

58 Mayo Foundation for Medical Education and Research, Special Report: Yoga and tai chi. Pathways to health and wholeness, October 2009, pp 1–8.

59 Frank JD: Common features of psychotherapy. Aust NZ J Psychiatry 1972;6:34–40.

60 Alarcón RD, Williams M: Cultural concepts in 'Persuasion and Healing'; in Alarcón RD, Frank JB (eds): The Psychotherapy of Hope. The Legacy of Persuasion and Healing. Baltimore, Johns Hopkins University Press, 2012, pp 88–106.

61 Mir G, Salway S, Kai J, Karlsen S, Bhopal R, Ellison GTH, Sheikh A: Principles for research on ethnicity and health. The Leeds Consensus Statement. Eur J Publ Health 2012. doi: 10.1093/europub/cks028.

62 Tseng WS: Culture and psychotherapy; in Teng WS, Streltzer J (eds): Cultural Competence in Clinical Psychiatry: Core Competencies in Psychotherapy. Washington, American Psychiatric Publishing, 2004, pp 181–198.

63 Calderón JL, Beltrán RA: Rethinking language and literacy for ensuring culturally appropriate health communication. Physicians Patients 2005;3:1–4.

64 Dyck E: Psychedelic Psychiatry. LSD from Clinic to Campus. Baltimore, Johns Hopkins University Press, 2008.

65 Collier D: Humphrey Osmond, Psychedelic Pioneer and the Doors of Perception. Montreal, Drawn & Quarterly Publications, 1988.

66 Markel H: An Anatomy of Addiction. Sigmund Freud, Sam Halsted, and the Miracle Drug Cocaine. New York, Pantheon Books, 2011.

67 Bennett D: Dr. Ecstasy. The New York Times Magazine, January 30, 2005, pp 30–37.

68 Breggin P: Brain Disabling Treatments in Psychiatry: Drugs, Electroshock and the Psychopharmaceutical Complex. New York, Springer, 2007.

69 Angell M: The Epidemic of Mental Illness: Why? The New York Rev Books, June 23, 2011, pp 20–22.

70 Angell M: The Illusions of Psychiatry. The New York Rev Books, July 14, 2011, pp 20–22.

71 Kirsch I: The Emperor's New Drugs: Exploding the Antidepressant Myth. New York, Basic Books, 2011.

72 Whitaker R: Anatomy of an Epidemic: Magic Bullets, Psychiatric Drugs, and the Astonishing Rise of Mental Illness in America. New York, Crown, 2011.

73 Hartzband P, Groopman J: Money and the changing culture of medicine. N Engl J Med 2009;360:221–227.

74 Oldham J: Letter to the Editor. New York Rev Books. August 18, 2011, p 82.

75 Stahl SM: Personalized Medicine, Pharmacogenomics, and the Practice of Psychiatry: On the Threshold of Predictive Therapeutics in Psychopharmacology? CNS Spectr 2008;13:115–118.

76 Ruiz P (ed): Ethnicity and Psychopharmacology. Washington, American Psychiatric Press, 2000.

77 Mrazek DA, Lerman C: Facilitating clinical implementation of pharmacogenomics (commentary). JAMA 2011;306:304–305.

78 Bradford D, Kim M, Braxton L, Marx C, Butterfield M: Access to medical care among persons with psychotic and major affective disorders. Psychiatr Serv 2008;59:847–850.

79 US Centers for Disease Control and Prevention Report: Mental Illness Surveillance Among Adults in the United States. Atlanta, 2011.

80 Mair F, Whitten P: Systematic review of studies of patient satisfaction with telemedicine. Br Med J 2000;320:1517–1520.

81 Mohr DC: Telemental health: reflections on how to move the field forward. Clin Psych Sci Pract 2009;16: 343–347.

82 Solnit R: A Paradise Built in Hell: The Extraordinary Communities that Arise in Disaster. New York, Viking, 2009.

83 Carey B: Expert on Mental Illness Reveals Her Own Fight. New York Times website http:www.nytimes.com/2011/06/23/health/23lives.html. Accessed June 23, 2011.

84 Institute of Medicine and National Research Council: Preventing mental, emotional and behavioral disorders among young people; in O'Connell ME, Boat T, Warner KE (eds): Progress and Possibilities. Washington, National Academies Press, 2009.

85 Ochsner KN, Bunge SA, Gross JJ, Gabrieli JD: Rethinking feelings: an fMRI study of the cognitive regulation of emotion. J Cognit Neurosci 2002;14:1215–1222.

86 Norris FH: Looking for resilience: understanding the longitudinal trajectories of responses to stress. Soc Sci Med 2009;21:90–96.

87 Southwick SM, Litz BT, Charney D, Friedman MJ (eds): Resilience and Mental Health Challenges Across the Lifespan. Cambridge, Cambridge University Press, 2011.

88 Chávez LM, Canino G, Negrón G, et al: Psychometric properties of the Spanish version of two mental health outcome measures: World Health Organization Disability Assessment Schedule II and Lehman's Quality of Life Interview. Ment Health Serv Res 2005;7:145–159.

89 Westen D: Discovering what works in the community: toward a genuine partnership of clinicians and researchers; in Hoffman SG, Weinberger J (eds): The Art and Science of Psychotherapy. New York, Routledge, 2007.

90 Geldard RG: Parmenides and the Way to Truth. Rhinebeck, Monkfish Books, 2007.

91 Bok S: Exploring Happiness: From Aristotle to Brain Science. New Haven, Yale University Press, 2010.

92 President's Council on Bioethics: Beyond Therapy: Biotechnology and the pursuit of Happiness. Washington, Regan Books, 2003.

93 McHugh PR, Slavney PR: The Perspectives of Psychiatry, ed 2. Baltimore, Johns Hopkins University Press, 1998.

94 Alarcón RD: Ambiguity at the crossroads of psychiatry and demoralization: reflections and possibilities. Eur J Psychiatry, 2013;in press.

95 Kirmayer LJ, Thombs BD, Jurcik T, Jarvis GE and Guzder J: Use of an expanded version of the DSM-IV outline for cultural formulation on a cultural consultation service. Psychiatr Serv 2008;59:683–686.

96 Bäärnhielm S, Scarpinati Rosso M: The cultural formulation: a model to combine nosology and patients life context in psychiatric diagnostic practice. Transcultural Psychiatry 2009;46:406–428.

97 Nagel T: Who Is Happy and When? The New York Rev Books, Dec 23, 2010, pp 46–48.

98 Mitchell L: Sick in the Head. Why America Won't Get the Health-Care System It Needs. Harper's Magazine, February 2009, pp 33–44.

Prof. Renato D. Alarcón, MD, MPH
Emeritus Professor of Psychiatry
Mayo Clinic College of Medicine, 200 First St. S.W.
Rochester, MN 55905 (USA)
E-Mail alarcon.renato@mayo.edu

Alarcón

Alarcón RD (ed): Cultural Psychiatry.
Adv Psychosom Med. Basel, Karger, 2013, vol 33, pp 15–30 (DOI: 10.1159/000348725)

Culture and Psychiatric Diagnosis

Roberto Lewis-Fernández[a, b] · Neil Krishan Aggarwal[a, b]

[a]Columbia University Department of Psychiatry and [b]New York State Psychiatric Institute,
New York, N.Y., USA

Abstract

Since the publication of DSM-IV in 1994, neurobiologists and anthropologists have criticized the rigidity of its diagnostic criteria that appear to exclude whole classes of alternate illness presentations, as well as the lack of attention in contemporary psychiatric nosology to the role of contextual factors in the emergence and characteristics of psychopathology. Experts in culture and mental health have responded to these criticisms by revising the very process of diagnosis for DSM-5. Specifically, the DSM-5 Cultural Issues Subgroup has recommended that concepts of culture be included more prominently in several areas: an introductory chapter on Cultural Aspects of Psychiatric Diagnosis – composed of a conceptual introduction, a revised Outline for Cultural Formulation, a Cultural Formulation Interview that operationalizes this Outline, and a glossary on cultural concepts of distress – as well as material directly related to culture that is incorporated into the description of each disorder. This chapter surveys these recommendations to demonstrate how culture and context interact with psychiatric diagnosis at multiple levels. A greater appreciation of the interplay between culture, context, and biology can help clinicians improve diagnostic and treatment planning. Copyright © 2013 APA*

The American Psychiatric Association (APA) released the 5th edition of the *Diagnostic and Statistical Manual of Mental Disorders* (DSM-5) in May of 2013 after revision efforts lasting nearly a decade. The various iterations of the DSM have been important documents for cultural psychiatry. The specified descriptions of mental disorders in these manuals fix the accepted phenomenological boundaries of diagnosable conditions. The goal of this specification is to standardize the definitions of disorders in order to guide research and clinical practice. However, an unintended consequence has been to exclude the alternative symptom variants of these disorders, which occur worldwide as a result of cultural and contextual factors [1].

In fact, the shift in emphasis after DSM-III to descriptively based assessment has resulted in less attention to several kinds of contextual information when making a diagnosis, not just cultural factors. By *context*, we refer to the social and environmental particularities of the local world in which individuals and groups develop. These elements include *culture* (e.g. meaning systems for interpreting human interactions and experiences more generally), *social structures* that constrain and allow diverse possibilities of activity and access to resources across individuals in a society (e.g. the health consequences of structural discrimination, such as racism), the *local material environment*, which sets the parameters for the group's engagement with natural resources and technology (e.g. the availability of certain medications in low-resource settings), as well as *individual circumstances*, which vary from person to person and over time. When applied to the diagnostic process, this cultural/contextual information includes the person's interpretation of the condition; whether it is considered pathological by others in the person's local setting; if pathological, what is the perceived level of severity; the dependence of the symptoms on particular situations or precipitants; and the relationship between the persistence of the disturbance and the availability or non-availability of supports and interventions [2]. In order to maximize the validity and usefulness of diagnosis, these cultural/contextual elements need to be included in the design and implementation of nosological systems.

Contemporary diagnostic manuals in psychiatry, however, have not pursued this approach. Over the last few decades, mental disorders have persistently been reduced to symptom lists devoid of contextual information. The circumstances that precipitate an emotional disturbance being assessed for major depressive disorder, for example, have become less important since the publication of DSM-III in 1980. By 1994, a patient presenting with 2 weeks of depressive symptoms could still be excluded from a DSM-IV diagnosis of major depressive disorder if the symptoms occurred within 2 months after a particular precipitant – the death of a loved one. The implication of this exclusion is that, in the context of bereavement, the emotional disturbance does not represent a pathological condition – despite sharing the same symptoms – but instead a normal grief reaction. In DSM-5, by contrast, this bereavement exclusion has been eliminated, and just meeting the symptom list will be sufficient for a diagnosis of major depressive disorder [3]. This almost exclusive reliance on clinical symptoms as the primary defining factors of the disorders argues for the importance of continuing to press for the inclusion of cultural and contextual factors in DSM-5.

This chapter summarizes key aspects of the work of and the recommendations from the DSM-5 Cultural Issues Subgroup, designed to improve the assessment of culture and context within psychiatric diagnosis. The Cultural Issues Subgroup was part of the larger Gender and Cross-Cultural Study Group and was composed of experts in cultural mental health. The subgroup was charged with making recommendations on racial, ethnic, cultural, and contextual issues to the all the work groups, such as differences in risk factors, precipitants, symptom presentations, prevalence, symptom severity, and course of illness. As part of this process, the subgroup organized literature reviews of relevant topics as well as a field trial in five continents of a newly developed Cultural Formulation Interview. Several of these literature reviews and field trial reports have been published and others will be forthcoming [4–7]. Specifically, the following recommendations for DSM-5 are reviewed: (1) a comprehensive introductory chapter that provides conceptual and practical guidance on evaluating the role of culture and context in diagnosis, and (2) culture-relevant material included in the descriptive text for each disorder. The introductory chapter would be composed of: (a) a conceptual introduction, (b) a slightly revised version of the DSM-IV Outline for Cultural Formulation, (c) the Cultural Formulation Interview, which operationalizes the Outline into a questionnaire, and (d) a glossary on cultural concepts of distress. It is important to acknowledge at the outset that this chapter was written as the content of DSM-5 was still under deliberation; therefore, it may also serve to document the interim history of the Subgroup and its interactions with other work groups and the DSM-5 leadership. Before describing the subgroup recommendations, however, we briefly review critiques from both neuroscience and anthropology related to specific diagnostic issues in DSM-IV.

Challenges of and to Diagnosis in DSM-5

Tasked with reviewing cultural content for the entire manual, the Cultural Issues Subgroup maintained a dual focus on two allied disciplines that strongly inform cultural psychiatry: cultural anthropology and neuroscience. These fields have challenged central tenets of diagnosis in DSM-IV and informed the revision process for DSM-5. A survey of criticisms from these fields lays a foundation to illustrate how culture and context relate to psychiatric diagnosis.

To begin, neurobiologists have raised concerns that are fundamental to the very act of diagnosis. They contend that current DSM-IV diagnoses are similar phenotypic expressions of different underlying mechanisms [8]. In the case of major depressive disorder, for example, only five symptoms are needed from a list of nine. In other words, two different major depressive disorder phenotypes can overlap only on one symptom [9]. They also question the use of binary categories in DSM-IV, even though the underlying psychopathology is most likely dimensional [8]. Disorders likely develop in degrees, not as a yes/no condition, and cutoff criteria are somewhat arbitrary based on few studies trying to predict long-term outcomes [10]. The categorical approach to diagnosis in DSM-IV may impede research exploring the relationship between neurobiology and the phenomenology of disorders, especially at sub-threshold levels [11]. Consequently, DSM-5 was expected to include dimensional aspects of disorders [12–16]. These debates, aimed at altering the process by which diagnoses are established in DSM-5, represented a notable departure from DSM-IV.

Anthropologists have also leveled substantial arguments against DSM-IV. They assert that psychiatrists have over-reified conditions based on the biomedical model, with the expectation of promoting research related to the biological factors of illness over social and cultural factors [17]. Psychiatrists have transformed reactions to adversity and complex dimensional experiences into fixed entities in conformity with the medical concept of disease. In contrast, anthropologists hold that many psychiatric conditions are more in the nature of reactions, experiences changing over time and place, with patterns of expression strongly determined by contextual factors that evolve historically. A reification of disorders mistakenly turns them into invariant diagnoses that ignore alternate possibilities of symptomatology. In addition, anthropologists dispute psychiatry's predominant focus on the individual, a particularly North Atlantic medical perspective that leads to locating pathology inside the person [18, 19]. This ignores the contributions of other health sciences, which show that social, cultural, and contextual determinants of health are equal if not more important contributors to psychopathology. This contextualization needs a place in clinical practice and research.

Both of these neurobiological and anthropological analyses point to a common direction: the current method of diagnosis in DSM-IV cannot account for varieties of illness presentations and experiences that lie outside of existing, categorical symptom criteria. Neurobiologists may wish for more precision at the levels of molecular biology, genetics, or functional neuroanatomy. Anthropologists may wish for more attention to research on the social and cultural etiologies, courses, and healing processes of illness. These perspectives are united by dissatisfaction with a diagnostic system that excludes subthreshold or alternate symptom expressions of mental disorders and that privileges descriptive, symptom-based approaches devoid of contextual information as the main way of defining psychopathology. As cultural psychiatrists, we believe that the relationship between biology and culture can be better understood through a greater examination of the contextual factors of illness. This tenet underlies the various proposals of the DSM-5 Cultural Issues Subgroup.

Principles Guiding Revisions on Culture and Diagnosis for DSM-5

In April 2010, the Cultural Issues Subgroup sent a memo to the DSM-5 leadership delineating how revisions relating to culture and psychiatric diagnosis can be integrated at several levels of the manual. A proposal written by Roberto Lewis-Fernández, Renato Alarcón, Laurence Kirmayer, and Kimberly Yonkers on behalf of all Subgroup members recommended inclusion of an introductory chapter on *Cultural Aspects of Psychiatric Diagnosis*. This chapter, to be preferably placed early and prominently in the manual, would provide a theoretical introduction to cultural issues in psychiatry. It would emphasize the value of cultural/contextual information as a way of enhancing diagnostic accuracy, and would include general instructions for use of the DSM-5 with patients from all cultural groups, but particularly those whose backgrounds may differ from those of their clinicians, as well as with immigrants, refugees, and in cases where the clinician felt uncertain about the nature of the information. The interview version of the DSM-IV Outline for Cultural Formulation and a glossary on cultural concepts of distress would furnish clinicians with methods to obtain this cultural/contextual information.

In drafting the proposal, members of the DSM-5 Cultural Issues Subgroup recalled experiences with DSM-IV in which culture appeared to be included as an afterthought to diagnosis [20]. For example, the APA accepted only a modified set of recommendations from the National Institute of Mental Health's Group on Culture and Diagnosis to enhance the cultural validity of DSM-IV. These modified recommendations included an introduction without definitions for race and ethnicity; a combined section on age, gender, and culture included in each disorder chapter, the Outline for Cultural Formulation placed in the next-to-last appendix, and a significantly shortened version of the Glossary of Culture-Bound Syndromes, also placed in the Appendix [19]. For DSM-5, the Cultural Issues Subgroup adopted an alternate approach: the centrality of culture within psychiatric diagnosis necessitates revisions that are implemented at all levels of the text. To draw upon spatial metaphors, these revisions can be seen as *horizontal* in that they infuse a cultural/contextual perspective to the manual as a whole as well as *vertical* in that they appear at various levels of the text.

Furthermore, the Cultural Issues Subgroup has operationalized theoretical developments from neurobiology and anthropology for clinical practice. For example, the need to account for social and cultural influences is reflected in the Subgroup's emphasis on ascertaining cultural/contextual information to increase diagnostic accuracy. In addition, cultural factors are posited as potential explanations for symptom variability of disorders based on their settings. Moreover, the Subgroup's Cultural Formulation Interview also utilizes a dimensional approach to assessment as an analogue to the dimensional approach for diagnosis.

The remainder of the chapter summarizes the subgroup recommendations. We will cover the proposed content of the introductory chapter first, followed by a brief description of how we suggested cultural/contextual information be included in the description of each disorder.

Introductory Chapter on Cultural Aspects of Psychiatric Diagnosis

Conceptual Introduction
The proposed draft of the introductory chapter began with the essential role of culture in diagnosis.

Understanding the cultural context of illness experience is essential for effective diagnostic assessment and clinical management. Mental disorders are defined in relation to social and cultural norms and values. Diagnostic assessment must therefore consider whether patients' experiences, symptoms, and behaviors differ from relevant sociocultural norms and lead to difficulties in adaptation in their cultures of origin and current social contexts. DSM-5 aims to help clinicians assess cultural features of clinical problems, and to support research on the influence of culture on mental health and illness.

This text begins to elaborate the Cultural Issues Subgroup's concept of the cultural/contextual approach. This perspective explicitly calls for situating mental disorders in relation to social and cultural norms and values. The conceptual introduction also provides a working definition of culture for clinicians. This definition is focused on the following characteristics of culture: how it touches all aspects of daily experience (e.g. knowledge, practices, language, family structures); the fact that it is learned and transmitted; how it organizes individual identities, interpersonal interactions, and social institutions; that cultures change over time and are open and dynamic; how individuals are exposed to multiple cultures, out of which individual identities and sense of experience are fashioned, and the need not to essentialize or stereotype cultures as unchanging.

Definitions of race and ethnicity were then provided as a contrast. These are related to racism and discrimination that results in health disparities, on the one hand, and to the development of cultural, ethnic, and racial identity on the other, which can be both a source of resilience as well as of 'psychological, interpersonal, and intergenerational conflict or difficulties in adaptation that require diagnostic assessment' (proposed DSM-5 text).

After providing these general definitions, the subgroup turned to the act of diagnosis. The text focused on how culture plays a key role in determining the level at which an experience becomes problematic or pathological. Cultural factors can result in the normalization of behaviors that may seem pathological in other contexts. For example, intensely shy, socially reticent behavior in certain cultural settings may be experienced by the person and seen by others as respectful, rather than as a sign of social anxiety disorder [21]. On the other hand, culture may also contribute to vulnerability and suffering, such as by amplifying fears that maintain panic disorder or health anxiety [22].

The draft text then focused on the cultural positioning of the DSM-5 itself.

As the distinction between mind, body, and spirit varies across cultures, the view that a problem is a mental disorder – as opposed to a physical illness or a social or moral predicament – depends on cultural modes of explanation and attribution. The DSM organizes disorders into broad categories (e.g. mood, anxiety, somatoform disorders) based on similarity in symptoms and putative underlying mechanisms. Across different cultural contexts, a problem may be organized differently on the basis of locally recognized symptoms and signs, presumed cause, course, or outcome. Furthermore, the correspondence between local culturally based nosology and DSM categories varies substantially. In general, there will be no one-to-one mapping of DSM and cultural categories; local nosology will provide additional information relevant to help-seeking, coping, and treatment expectations.

This conceptual introduction asserts that culture belongs to everyone, not just underserved or unfamiliar racial or ethnic minorities from a given society. Culture also frames the entire experience of mental health and illness for the patient and the clinician. For patients, culture molds the interpretations of thoughts, emotions, and behaviors that rise to the level of symptoms. Culture also influences the types and ways of seeking help. For clinicians, culture supplies the general assumptions and structural divisions of psychiatric classifications. In this way, diagnosis inherently represents a cross-cultural exercise given the possibility that patients and clinicians may not share the same understandings of illness.

The introduction is meant to orient clinicians to the relationship between culture and diagnosis. Within this framework, the Cultural Issues Subgroup also provided tangible methods to increase cultural/contextual validity. The Cultural Formulation Interview exemplifies one approach.

Outline for Cultural Formulation and Cultural Formulation Interview

The Cultural Formulation Interview (CFI) is a DSM-5 innovation. It operationalizes the DSM-IV Outline for Cultural Formulation (OCF) into a set of questions and explicit instructions. The main goal of the OCF in DSM-IV was to help clinicians identify cultural-contextual factors affecting the patient that are relevant to diagnosis and treatment [23]. The OCF organized the relevance of culture within the patient-clinician encounter around five dimensions: (1) the cultural identity of the individual, (2) the cultural explanations of the individual's illness, (3) the cultural factors related to psychosocial environment and levels of functioning, (4) cultural elements of the relationship between the individual and the clinicians, and (5) the overall cultural assessment for diagnosis and care [24, 25]. An explicit function of the OCF has been to assist clinicians in diagnosing patients whose presentations do not correspond to DSM-IV diagnoses [17, 20]. An OCF composed of the same five dimensions was edited for comprehensiveness, clarity, and length (e.g. addition of other elements of cultural identity such as religious affiliation and sexual orientation).

The OCF has been called the most important contribution of anthropology to psychiatry [17, 26]. Journals such as *Culture, Medicine and Psychiatry* and *Transcultural Psychiatry* have regularly published cases on the benefits of its incorporation in mental health assessment. The OCF has been widely used within psychiatric education to impart cultural competency among trainees [27]. However, it has been criticized on several fronts: busy clinicians may not use it if it takes too much time [28], its dimensions may be too indistinct and overlapping [29], and use of the OCF may repeat information from the standard clinical assessment [30]. The Cultural Issues Subgroup has counted at least four versions of the OCF whose different formats may prevent the standardization of training and research [31]. Nonetheless, researchers from McGill University found that culture has a significant impact on psychiatric diagnosis through their use of the OCF within a cultural consultation service. Among a total of 323 patients referred over a 10-year period, 34 (49%) of 70 cases with a referral diagnosis of a psychotic disorder were rediagnosed as having a nonpsychotic disorder and 12 (5%) of the 253 cases with a referral diagnosis of a nonpsychotic disorder were rediagnosed as having a psychotic disorder [32]. These results demonstrated that the OCF is a useful adjunct to diagnosis and deserved further revisions to facilitate its use.

In light of these developments, the Cultural Issues Subgroup formed an international consortium of research collaborators to develop and test the CFI, a standardized 16-item questionnaire that operationalizes the OCF. The questions are intended for use at the beginning of a routine mental health evaluation and cover the same topical areas as the OCF. The CFI includes instructions that precede the questions and a guide to the interviewer on the type of content that can be generated by each question. It is organized into four sections: (1) cultural definition of the problem (questions 1–3), (2) cultural perceptions of cause, context, and support (questions 4–10), (3) cultural factors affecting self-coping and past help seeking (questions 11–13), and (4) cultural factors affecting current help seeking (questions 14–16).

In order to avoid stereotyping, the CFI is personalized in that it focuses on the views of the individual patient, rather than inquiring generically about the views of the group(s) the person self-identifies with or is ascribed to by the clinician [2]. This allows the intracultural heterogeneity of views to emerge. It also accounts for hybrid identities in the person, since individuals typically hold views that stem from a diversity of cultural influences in their life, which can best be assessed on an individual basis [33]. To facilitate this use of the CFI, the concept of culture that informs the CFI is composed of the following three elements:

(a) The values, orientations, knowledge, and practices that individuals derive from membership in diverse social groups (e.g. ethnic groups, faith communities, occupational groups, and veterans).

(b) Aspects of a person's background that may affect his or her perspective, such as geographical origin, migration, language, religion, sexual orientation, or race/ethnicity.

(c) The influence of family, friends, and other community members (the person's *social network*) on the person's illness experience (proposed DSM-5 text).

Cultural factors are subordinated to the information that can be elicited from individual patients, including their perspectives on the views of their social group.

Another aspect of the CFI that bears noting is that it is not intended exclusively for the evaluation of members of nondominant cultural groups, such as racial/ethnic minorities. Instead, the CFI is intended for use by any clinician with any patient in any setting. Patients and clinicians who appear to share the same cultural background may nevertheless differ in ways that are relevant to care. At the same time, the CFI instructions suggest useful settings and patient-clinician matches, such as:

…when there is difficulty in diagnostic assessment, owing to significant differences in the cultural, religious, or socioeconomic backgrounds of clinician and patient; when there is uncertainty about the fit between culturally expressed symptoms and diagnostic criteria; when it is difficult to judge illness severity or impairment; when patient and clinician disagree on the course of care, or in cases of limited treatment engagement and adherence.

Thus, the main goals of the CFI are to enhance the cultural validity of diagnostic assessment, facilitate treatment planning, and promote patient engagement. The CFI

Lewis-Fernández · Krishan Aggarwal

can be seen as operationalizing aspects of culture presented in the conceptual introduction. In particular, clinicians are encouraged to detect discrepancies in symptom presentation against DSM criteria, uncertainties in illness severity and impairment, differences of opinion on the course of care, and how clinician identities may interact with patient identities throughout the evaluation. The ascertainment of cultural/contextual information comprises an essential step of the diagnostic process and the CFI is an evidence-based method of obtaining this information. However, the CFI by itself does not result in a diagnosis. The information it obtains must be integrated with other available clinical material to produce a comprehensive clinical and contextual evaluation. Not only the information elicited by the CFI but also the process of conducting the Interview is expected to be helpful in this regard. Better patient engagement, for example, may result as much from greater diagnostic validity resulting from the information obtained as from the patient's perception of being attended to and understood – a fact that comes mostly from the patient-centered nature of the CFI items. Which aspect of the CFI is useful for which outcome is a topic for further studies.

As part of the development of the CFI for DSM-5 an APA-supported field trial was conducted. With a targeted enrollment of 330 patients in six countries across five continents, the field trial attempted to test the feasibility (can it be done?), acceptability (do people like it?), and perceived clinical utility (is it helpful?) of the CFI among patients and clinicians. Data on the first 200 patients was used to revise the initial version of the CFI into the final version to be included in DSM-5. Final field data results will be available in mid-2013.

In addition, eleven supplementary modules to be used in conjunction with the CFI have been created to further help clinicians conduct a more comprehensive cultural assessment for patients who require it. Topical modules cover explanatory models, level of functioning, influence of social network on illness course, psychosocial and economic stressors, role of spirituality, religion, and moral traditions, cultural identity, coping and help seeking, and the patient-clinician relationship. Population-specific modules address the special needs of school-age children and adolescents, older adults, immigrants and refugees, and caregivers. Clinicians may choose to utilize all modules for a full assessment or apply selected modules if they wish to expand a particular component of the CFI.

Glossary of Cultural Concepts of Distress
The Cultural Issues Subgroup proposed a thorough revision of the DSM-IV *Glossary of Culture-Bound Syndromes* into a new *Glossary of Cultural Concepts of Distress* to be included in the introductory chapter. The new Glossary substitutes the older formulation of *culture-bound syndromes* with three concepts of greater clinical utility.

Cultural syndromes are clusters of symptoms and attributions that tend to co-occur among individuals in specific cultural groups, communities, or contexts and that are recognized locally as coherent patterns of experience. *Cultural idioms of distress* are ways of expressing distress that may not involve specific symptoms or syndromes, but that provide shared ways of experiencing and talking about personal or social concerns (e.g. everyday talk about 'nerves' or 'depression'). *Cultural explanations* or *perceived causes* are labels, attributions, or features of an explanatory model that indicate culturally recognized meaning or etiology for symptoms, illness, or distress [5, 34, 35] (proposed DSM-5 text).

Although worth distinguishing conceptually, in common practice the same cultural term frequently denotes more than one kind of cultural concept. A familiar example of this usage may be the concept of 'depression', which can describe a syndrome (e.g. major depressive disorder), an idiom of distress (e.g. as in the common expression 'I feel depressed'), or a perceived cause (similar to 'stress'). Despite this overlap, the distinctions between syndromes, idioms, and causes can help clinicians recognize how cultural concepts are deployed by patients and thus facilitate diagnosis and treatment negotiation. The glossary provided nine examples of cultural concepts of distress from around the world typifying syndromes, idioms, causes and their inter-relationships. Only high-prevalence concepts that have received considerable research attention are included, and for each concept, the glossary lists the related psychiatric diagnoses. These examples are intended to assist clinicians in the evaluation and treatment of individuals who present for care reporting these nine specific cultural concepts, but they are also meant to illustrate the process by which providers can translate from local expressions to DSM diagnoses.

In fact, the glossary devotes considerable attention to explaining the relationship of cultural concepts to the conventional diagnoses in the body of the manual. One way to understand the cultural concepts presented in the glossary is that many DSM disorders started out as local expressions which over time became operationalized prototypes of disorder, based on a process of abstraction and generalization. Yet these prototypes do not exhaust cultural diversity in presentation, not only for cultural expressions that are closely related to DSM diagnoses (e.g. alternate versions of panic attacks), but especially for entirely different ways of organizing the classification of psychopathology (e.g. alternate types of disorder, such as anger-related conditions). As a result, clinicians may be exposed to local phenomena of distress that do not conform easily to conventional diagnoses. In fact, most of the cultural concepts included in the glossary cut across DSM diagnoses, so that the relationship between concepts and disorders is not one-to-one, but instead one-to-many in either direction [36]. Symptoms or behaviors that might be sorted by DSM-5 into several disorders may be included in a single folk concept, and diverse presentations that might be classified by DSM-5 as variants of a single disorder may be sorted into several distinct concepts by an indigenous diagnostic system. In effect, the existence of these alternate presentations suggests that *all* forms of distress are locally shaped [36].

In order to deliver culturally appropriate care, it can be very useful to understand the association between locally patterned differences in symptoms, ways of talking about distress, and locally perceived causes, on the one hand, and coping strategies and patterns of help-seeking, on the other. Therefore, the Glossary clarifies and illustrates the various ways in which knowledge of the cultural grounding of cultural concepts of distress can be important to diagnostic practice and clinical care in general. These were included to avoid misdiagnosis, to obtain clinically useful information, to improve rapport and engagement, to improve therapeutic efficacy, to guide clinical research, and to clarify the cultural epidemiology.

Culture-Relevant Material Included in the Descriptive Text for Each Disorder

The sections above summarized the proposed DSM-5 revisions that address what we have called a *horizontal* approach to infusing a cultural/contextual perspective to the manual as a whole. The following section covers the recommendations that we have labeled *vertical*, that is, they appear in each disorder chapter at various levels of the text. While the DSM-IV limited the explicitly culture-related material for each disorder to a single section on Specific Culture, Age, and Gender Features, the DSM-5 separates this section into three independent sections on Development Culture, and Gender. Some work groups took this opportunity to pursue a comprehensive revision of cultural factors relevant to each disorder. In the interest of space, we illustrate this approach with examples from the work group on Anxiety, Obsessive-Compulsive Spectrum, Posttraumatic, and Dissociative Disorders.

The first step in this more comprehensive approach was to review the quality of the existing data on cultural variations for each DSM-IV disorder in order to recommend revisions for DSM-5. This involved answering the following questions: For each disorder, what level of integration is needed for cultural information within DSM-5? Is the evidence strong enough to warrant changes to disorder criteria? Or, instead, should cultural data go only in the descriptive text to help the clinician apply existing criteria across cultural presentations? Alternatively, should nothing be changed from DSM-IV? The basis for this approach is the view that every disorder description is incomplete until it includes the full range of cultural variations of the syndrome worldwide. Clearly, an institutionalized process with multiple stakeholders, such as the DSM revisions, is inherently resistant to change, sometimes appropriately so. It can be destabilizing, for example, to make too many changes at once in a nosology that has clinical, social, forensic, and fiscal implications. Not only these sociopolitical processes but also the shortcomings of the existing datasets limited the extent of cultural variation that could be proposed. Yet, within these constraints, the work group marshaled the evidence for change.

Sometimes, the data were robust enough to warrant proposed revisions at the level of criteria sets. This was the case for social anxiety disorder, agoraphobia, specific phobia, posttraumatic stress disorder, and dissociative identity disorder, among others. Social anxiety disorder may serve as an example [37]. Decades of cross-cultural research have noted that the fear of negative evaluation by others, which is the hallmark of this disorder, can take the form of fear that the individual will offend others, in addition to or instead of the fear that the person will feel embarrassed or humiliated as a result of engaging in the social behavior [38, 39]. Labeled 'other-directed' or 'allocentric' fear, this type of fear is a characteristic symptom of certain forms of culturally described distress in East Asia, such as *taijin kyofusho* in Japan and *taein kong po* in Korea. However, fear of offending others is also observed among individuals with social anxiety disorder in many cultural settings, such as Australia and the US [39, 40]. In fact, in many cases cross-culturally, the fear of offending others and the fear of embarrassment or humiliation occur together, rather than being mutually exclusive, indicating that they are related presentations [37]. The work group felt that the cross-cultural evidence was sufficiently robust to revise social anxiety disorder criteria to indicate this relationship, which is intended to help reduce misdiagnosis in settings where 'other-directed' fear is the primary or initial presentation. The revised social anxiety disorder criterion B would now read: 'The individual fears that he or she will act in a way or show anxiety symptoms that will be negatively evaluated (e.g. be humiliated, embarrassed, rejected, *or offend others*)' (italics added) (proposed DSM-5 text).

At other times, evidence on the impact of cultural factors in diagnosis was not felt to warrant a revision of diagnostic criteria but was considered a useful addition to the fuller description of the disorder, e.g. its diagnostic features, associated features, and prevalence. The intent was to help clinicians and researchers identify individuals suffering from the disorder and facilitate assessments of severity, comorbidity, and prognosis as well as treatment options. Cultural contributions to the text took several forms:

(a) In light of the growing international use of the DSM revisions, an effort was made throughout the text to limit its ethnocentricity. Clear notation was made of the geographic and cultural origin of the data provided. For example, under the section for prevalence, data reported US racial/ethnic, and international variation. If studies were only available from certain regions of the world (e.g. the US and Europe), this was noted in the relevant sections of the disorder chapter, e.g. under Risk and Prognostic Factors. The goal is to advance toward a truly international nosology that can more easily be integrated with ICD-11. A first step is to clarify the limitations of the existing data; if most of the information comes from only a few geographic regions, this raises the question of its generalizability and also identifies the logical next areas for research.

(b) Two sections of the text, those on diagnostic features and on prevalence, included culture-relevant information directly. The former described any symptom variation in the clinical presentation that led to a revision of disorder criteria, i.e. the social anxiety disorder revision of criterion B mentioned above. The section on Prevalence included prevalence variation by race/ethnicity in the US and the range of prevalence internationally. For example, most of the anxiety disorders have been examined in many countries with the same instrument, the Composite International

Diagnostic Interview, yielding comparable 12-month prevalence. The values from countries with the highest and lowest estimates of prevalence were reported as the endpoints of a range for each disorder.

(c) The rest of the cultural material went into a dedicated section on *Culture-Related Diagnostic Issues*. This section calls for comprehensive evaluation of local expressions of each disorder by including assessment of cultural concepts of distress, and contained most of the data on explicitly culture-related aspects of each disorder, such as on cultural variation in disorder symptoms that did not warrant criterial revision, as well as in development and course of the disorder, risk and prognostic factors, interpretation of stressors, impairment, and severity. More fine-grained information on cultural, racial, or ethnic variations in disorder prevalence (e.g. by nativity status, or subethnicity) was included in this section. Finally, information on cultural labels, explanatory models, or cultural syndromes associated with the disorder were included here and cross-referenced with individual entries in the *Glossary of Cultural Concepts of Distress* in the introductory chapter. An example is the complex association between *ataques de nervios* (attacks of nerves), a cultural syndrome common among Latinos, and several DSM-5 disorders [4, 41]. Individual presentations of *ataque* can be variously diagnosed as panic disorder, other specified dissociative disorder, and functional neurologic symptom (conversion) disorder, among others. That is, the cultural label unifies presentations that are considered psychiatrically diverse.

As an example of the kind of material that has been proposed for the explicit 'culture-related' section of each disorder chapter, we can consider posttraumatic stress disorder. This section includes information on variations in the risk of onset and severity of posttraumatic stress disorder as a result of various cultural/contextual factors. Examples of these factors are: variation in the type of traumatic exposure (e.g. genocide), the impact on disorder severity of the meaning attributed to the traumatic event (e.g. inability to perform funerary rites after a mass killing), the ongoing sociocultural context (e.g. residing among unpunished perpetrators in postconflict settings), and other cultural factors (e.g. acculturative stress in immigrants) [42]. The section also notes that the clinical expression of the individual symptoms or symptom clusters of posttraumatic stress disorder may vary culturally, particularly with respect to avoidance and numbing symptoms, distressing dreams, and somatic symptoms (e.g. dizziness, shortness of breath, heat sensations) [42–45]. Other information in this section includes the role that cultural syndromes and idioms of distress play in the expression of posttraumatic stress disorder and in the range of comorbid disorders. Thus, cultural concepts of distress provide behavioral and cognitive templates that link traumatic exposures to specific symptoms [5]. For example, panic attack symptoms may be salient in posttraumatic stress disorder among Cambodians and Latin Americans due to the association of traumatic exposure with panic-like *khyâl* attacks and *ataque de nervios* [42].

Conclusion

This chapter has summarized many of the proposals from the DSM-5 Cultural Issues Subgroup that relate to the role of culture and context in psychiatric diagnosis. The subgroup has taken into account the recommendations of neurobiologists and anthropologists who have criticized the rigidity of DSM-IV diagnostic criteria that exclude alternate illness presentations and that do not account for the role of context in the emergence and characteristics of psychopathology. The subgroup's revisions can be conceptualized horizontally as a cultural/contextual orientation throughout the entire Manual and vertically as a collection of revisions at various levels of the text. These recommendations include an introductory chapter on Cultural Aspects of Psychiatric Diagnosis – composed of a conceptual introduction, the revised Outline for Cultural Formulation, a Cultural Formulation Interview that operationalizes this outline, and a glossary on cultural concepts of distress – as well as material directly related to culture and incorporated into the description of each disorder. The intent of these revisions is to enhance the validity and reliability of psychiatric diagnosis across cultural groups in the United States and around the world.

Acknowledgments

The authors express their appreciation for the work of all their colleagues on the Cultural Issues Subgroup of the DSM-5 Gender and Culture Study Group, their international collaborators on the Cultural Formulation Interview field trial, and their colleagues on other DSM-5 work groups. We are also grateful for the support of the staff of the New York State Center of Excellence for Cultural Competence at New York State Psychiatric Institute. Special thanks to Andel Nicasio, Marit Boiler, and Ravi de Silva.

References

1 Kleinman A: Rethinking Psychiatry: From Cultural Category to Personal Experience. New York, Free Press, 1988.

2 Kleinman A, Benson P: Anthropology in the clinic: the problem of cultural competency and how to fix it. PLoS Medicine 2006;3:e294.

3 Zisook S, Shear K, Kendler KS: Validity of the bereavement exclusion criterion for the diagnosis of major depressive episode. World Psychiatry 2007;6:102–107.

4 Lewis-Fernández R, Guarnaccia PJ, Martínez IE, Salmán E, Schmidt A, Liebowitz M: Comparative phenomenology of ataques de nervios, panic attacks, and panic disorder. Cult Med Psychiatry 2002;26:199–223.

5 Hinton DE, Lewis-Fernández R: Idioms of distress among trauma survivors: Subtypes and clinical utility. Cult Med Psychiatry 2010;34:209–218.

6 Spiegel D, Loewenstein RJ, Lewis-Fernández R, Sar V, Simeon D, Vermetten E, Cardeña E, Dell PF: Redefining dissociative disorders for DSM-5. Depr Anx 2011;28:824–852.

7 Brown RJ, Lewis-Fernández R: Culture and conversion disorder: implications for DSM-5. Psychiatry Interpers Biol Proc 2011;74:187–206.

8 Hyman SE: Can neuroscience be integrated into the DSM-V? Nat Rev Neurosci 2007;8:725–732.

9 Kendler KS, Neale MC, Kessler RC, Heath AC, Eaves LJ: Major depression and generalized anxiety disorder: same genes, (partly) different environments? Arch Gen Psychiatry 1992;49:716–722.

10 Brown TA, Barlow DH: A proposal for a dimensional classification system based on the shared features of the DSM-IV anxiety and mood disorders: implications for assessment and treatment. Psychol Assess 2009;21:256–271.

11 Insel TR, Cuthbert B, Garvey M, Heinssen R, Pine DS, Quinn K, Sanislow C, Wang P: Research Domain Criteria (RDoC): toward a new classification framework for research on mental disorders. Am J Psychiatry 2010;167:748–751.

12 Goldberg D, Simms LJ, Gater R, Krueger RF: Integration of dimensional spectra for depression and anxiety into categorical diagnoses for general medical practice; in Regier DA, Narrow WE, Kuhl EA, Kupfer DJ (eds): The Conceptual Evolution of DSM-5. Arlington, American Psychiatric Publishing, 2011, pp 19–36.

13 Frank E, Rucci P, Cassano GB: One way forward for psychiatric nomenclature: the example of the spectrum project approach; in Regier DA, Narrow WE, Kuhl EA, Kupfer DJ (eds): The Conceptual Evolution of DSM-5. Arlington, American Psychiatric Publishing, 2011, pp 37–58.

14 Helzer JE: A proposal for incorporating clinically relevant dimensions into DSM-5; in Regier DA, Narrow WE, Kuhl EA, Kupfer DJ (eds): The Conceptual Evolution of DSM-5. Arlington, American Psychiatric Publishing, 2011, pp 81–96.

15 Krueger RF, Eaton NR, South SC, Clark LA, Simms LJ: Empirically derived personality disorder prototypes: Bridging dimensions and categories in DSM-5; in Regier DA, Narrow WE, Kuhl EA, Kupfer DJ (eds): The Conceptual Evolution of DSM-5. Arlington, American Psychiatric Publishing, 2011, pp 97–118.

16 Wittchen HU, Höfler M, Gloster AT, Craske MG, Beesda K. Options and dilemmas of dimensional measures for DSM-5: which types of measures fare best in predicting course and outcome? In Regier DA, Narrow WE, Kuhl EA, Kupfer DJ (eds): The Conceptual Evolution of DSM-5. Arlington, American Psychiatric Publishing, 2011, pp 119–144.

17 Good BJ: Culture and DSM-IV: diagnosis, knowledge and power. Cult Med Psychiatry 1996;20:127–132.

18 Littlewood R: Against pathology: the new psychiatry and its critics. Br J Psychiatry 1991;159:696–702.

19 Mezzich JE, Kirmayer LJ, Kleinman A, Fabrega H Jr, Parron DL, Good BJ, Lin KM, Manson SM: The place of culture in DSM-IV. J Nerv Ment Dis 1999; 187:457–464.

20 Lewis-Fernández R, Díaz N: The cultural formulation: a method for assessing cultural factors affecting the clinical encounter. Psychiatr Q 2002;73:271–295.

21 Heinrichs N, Rapee RM, Alden LA, Bögels S, Hofmann SG, Oh KJ, Sakano Y: Cultural differences in perceived social norms and social anxiety. Behav Res Ther 2006;44:1187–1197.

22 Hinton DE, Lewis-Fernández R, Pollack MH: A model of the generation of *ataque de nervios*: the role of fear of negative affect and fear of arousal symptoms. CNS Neurosci Ther 2009;15:264–275.

23 Mezzich JE, Caracci G, Fabrega H, Kirmayer LJ: Cultural formulation guidelines. Transcult Psychiatry 2009;46:383–405.

24 Lu FG, Lim RF, Mezzich JE: Issues in the assessment and diagnosis of culturally diverse individuals. Am Psychiatr Press Rev Psychiatry 1995;14:477–510.

25 Lewis-Fernández R: Cultural formulation of psychiatric diagnosis. Cult Med Psychiatry 1996;20:133–144.

26 Jenkins J: Anthropology and psychiatry: the contemporary convergence; in Bhugra D, Bhui K (eds): Textbook of Cultural Psychiatry. Cambridge, Cambridge University Press, 2007, pp 20–32.

27 Aggarwal NK, Rohrbaugh R: Teaching cultural competency through an experiential seminar on anthropology and psychiatry. Acad Psychiatry 2011;35: 331–334.

28 Lewis-Fernández R: The cultural formulation. Transcult Psychiatry 2009;46:379–382.

29 Ton H, Lim RF: The assessment of culturally diverse individuals; in Lim RF (ed): Clinical Manual of Cultural Psychiatry. Arlington, American Psychiatric Publishing, 2006, pp 3–31.

30 Caballero Martínez L: DSM-IV-TR cultural formulation of psychiatric cases: two proposals for clinicians. Transcult Psychiatry 2009;46:506–523.

31 Alarcón RD: Culture, cultural factors and psychiatric diagnosis: review and projections. World Psychiatry 2009;8:131–139.

32 Adeponle AB, Thombs BD, Groleau D, Jarvis E, Kirmayer LJ: Using the cultural formulation to resolve uncertainty in diagnoses of psychosis among ethnoculturally diverse patients. Psychiatr Serv 2012;63: 147–153.

33 Aggarwal NK: Hybridity and intersubjectivity in the clinical encounter: Impact on the cultural formulation. Transcult Psychiatry 2012;49:121–139.

34 Groleau D, Young A, Kirmayer LJ: The McGill Illness Narrative Interview (MINI): an interview schedule to elicit meanings and modes of reasoning related to illness experience. Transcult Psychiatry 2006;43:671–691.

35 Nicther M: Idioms of distress: alternatives in the expression of psychosocial distress: a case study from South India. Cult Med Psychiatry 1981;5:379–408.

36 Kleinman A: How is culture important for DSM-IV?; In Mezzich JE, Kleinman A, Fábrega H, Parron DL (eds): Culture and Psychiatric Diagnosis: a DSM-IV Perspective. Washington, American Psychiatric Press, 1996, pp 15–25.

37 Lewis-Fernández R, Hinton DE, Laria AJ, Patterson EH, Hofmann SG, Craske MG, Stein DJ, Asnaani A, Liao B: Culture and the anxiety disorders: recommendations for DSM-V. Depr Anx 2010;27:212–229.

38 Kirmayer L: The place of culture in psychiatric nosology: taijin kyofusho and DSM-III-R. J Nerv Ment Dis 1991;179:19–28.

39 Choy Y, Schneier F, Heimberg R, et al: Features of the offensive subtype of Taijin-Kyofu-Sho in US and Korean patients with DSMIV social anxiety disorder. Depr Anx 2008;25:230–240.

40 Kim J, Rapee R, Ja Oh K, Moon H: Retrospective report of social withdrawal during adolescence and current maladjustment in young adulthood: cross-cultural comparisons between Australian and South Korean students. J Adolesc 2008;31:543–563.

41 Guarnaccia PJ, Rivera M, Franco F, Neighbors C: The experiences of ataques de nervios: towards an anthropology of emotions in Puerto Rico. Cult Med Psychiatry 1996;20:343–367.

42 Hinton DE, Lewis-Fernández R: The cross-cultural validity of posttraumatic stress disorder: implications for DSM-5. Depr Anx 2011;28:783–801.

43 Hinton DE, Hinton A, Chhean D, et al: Nightmares among Cambodian refugees: the breaching of concentric ontological security. Cult Med Psychiatry 2009b;33:219–265.

44 Kirmayer LJ, Sartorius N: Cultural models and somatic syndromes. Psychosom Med 2007;69:832–840.

45 McCall GJ, Resick PA: A pilot study of PTSD symptoms among Kalahari Bushmen. J Trauma Stress 2003;16:445–450.

Roberto Lewis-Fernández, MD
New York State Psychiatric Institute
1051 Riverside Drive, Suite 3200, Unit 69
New York, NY 10032 (USA)
E-Mail rlewis@nyspi.columbia.edu

Alarcón RD (ed): Cultural Psychiatry.
Adv Psychosom Med. Basel, Karger, 2013, vol 33, pp 31–39 (DOI: 10.1159/000348727)

Trends in Cultural Psychiatry in the United Kingdom

Kamaldeep Bhui

Wolfson Institute of Preventive Medicine, Barts and London School of Medicine and Dentistry,
Queen Mary University of London, London, UK

Dedicated to Wen-Shing Tseng 1935–2012.
Professor of Psychiatry at University of Hawaii.
Founding President of the World Association of Cultural Psychiatry.

Abstract

Cultural psychiatry in the United Kingdom exhibits unique characteristics closely related to its history as a colonial power, its relationship with Commonwealth countries and the changing sociodemographic characteristics of its diverse population throughout the centuries. It is not surprising, therefore, that the emergence of this discipline was centred around issues of race and religion. After a brief historical review of the development of cultural psychiatry and the mention of pioneering intellectual and academic figures, as well as the evolvement of the field in organizations such as the Royal College of Psychiatrists, this chapter examines the need of a critical cultural psychiatry, more than a narrative social science distanced from the realities of clinical practice. In such context, issues such as policies and experience with efforts to delivering race equality, and address inequities in a renewed public health approach seem to confer British cultural psychiatry with a defined socially active role aimed at the pragmatic management, understanding and improvement of diverse and alternative systems of care and care practices.

Cultural psychiatry has become a popular subject of interest amongst experienced and trainee psychiatrists in the United Kingdom, but it has not always been that way. The UK does not have a separate organisation or faculty of cultural psychiatry, perhaps reflecting the way in which the country considers culture as an unclear and indistinct although relevant construct compared to others encountered by psychiatrists, i.e. what is cultural and what is social. Clearly, the collective beliefs and practices of distinct groups defining their identity through those beliefs (be they tribal, ethnic, race, or religious) are a subset of wider social factors and beliefs that can influence health and well-being. But why has cultural psychiatry become more popular in the UK, yet not as popular as in other countries?

The UK's history as a colonial power, the sustained relationship with Commonwealth countries, and the generations of migrants from former colonies has recently been overtaken by in-migration from the European Union. Each of these waves of migration have introduced new peoples to the UK and British traditions and ways of life, not to mention exposure of new migrants to the British social, health, educational and political systems. The relevance of these waves of immigration and the historical links with countries around the world is that people from these countries have shaped ideas in the UK about what constitutes culture, mainly thought of as an issue of migration and immigrants, ethnic differences, religious diversity, and race-related influences.

Consequently, unlike the USA, Canada or Australia where there are more or less large groups of indigenous peoples, or other countries which have seen little migration until recently, the UK notion of cultural psychiatry has been one of assessing, diagnosing and treating people who are different, in terms of their cultural heritage (meaning race, ethnicity, or religion or language or country of origin,) from that of the clinician. Most importantly, in the UK, the emergence of cultural psychiatry is centred around issues of race and religion, the two most conspicuous ways of classifying the patient to be different from the professional. Yet even this has changed, as the health service workforce has been made up, until recently, of migrants from the Commonwealth countries, and more recently from East Europe and Europe in general. Despite the heavy exposure to diverse cultures, languages, religions and races the British health and social care system do still aim to treat all people as the same; in fact, there seem to be some fears about overstating or emphasising differences which can become politically and socially divisive. The recent debates in the UK about multi-culturalism being responsible for terrorism exemplify this dilemma.

The subjects of clinical relevance and interest taken up by cultural psychiatrists in the UK include clinical and research investigations of immigrants and migrants, this includes the plight of asylum seekers and refugees, initially focused on black people of Caribbean and African origin, people from the Indian sub-continent including India, Bangladesh and Pakistan. Other immigrant groups such as those from China, Vietnam, or European countries have not yet received as much research attention. Indeed, the Irish have not received as much attention either, but their health indices, are poorer than the White English groups. Other areas of interest have included racism and discrimination, the relationship between religion and mental health and, more recently, the organisation and delivery of health services for diverse populations, and the training of psychiatrists to ensure they are culturally competent. This latter interest is itself bedevilled by controversy about what is cultural competence, who needs the training, and whether the real issue is workforce representation, the responsibility of training organisations and employers not clinicians. The narrow focus on ethnic minorities that are visible in the UK is mostly sustained by arguments of clinical relevance, so that a wider understanding of culture and its influence on mental health and well-being, as well as mental disorders, is not adequately considered.

Cultural psychiatry in USA and Canada has been largely influenced by anthropology. Although similar influences are found in the UK, as exemplified by the seminal work of John Cox, Roland Littlewood and Maurice Lipsedge, anthropology has not been a dominant factor; it has been rather a 'critical friend' of sociology, psychology, history, health services research and public health sciences. There have even been movements such as critical psychiatry and social perspectives in psychiatry. Each of these has recently attempted to challenge the power relationships established in a culturally blind approach to assessing, diagnosing and treating mental illness. Thus, cultural psychiatry in the UK involves a number of commentators, disciplines and approaches reflecting the needs of clinicians and trainees, but also the priorities of the experts in cultural psychiatry. It can also be said that the priorities and pragmatic expectations of the majority of clinicians include viewing cultural psychiatry as a way of improving the outcome for patients who are different from themselves in terms of language, race or ethnicity.

Brief Historical Review

Among the pioneers of cultural psychiatry in the UK, the name of Phillip Rack stands out. In the 1980s, he set up the Transcultural Psychiatry Unit in Bradford, a community in the industrial North of England which faced an economic decline; Bradford has a large Pakistani population which has remained rather isolated and insular, leading to fears about conflict with the wider public. Rack tackled both cultural and religious beliefs and influences of the local immigrant population as well as the way services needed to be adapted to its needs.

John Cox edited one of the earliest British textbooks on the topic, titled precisely *Transcultural Psychiatry*, and published in 1986 [1]. The authors' list included all the impressive and influential thinkers who were able to see and study cultural impacts on assessment, diagnosis and treatment, and to demonstrate that some people did not benefit from the 'one size fits all' paradigm that psychiatric research and practice has sought to evidence. Such authors include H.B.M. Murphy, Julian Leff, John Bavington, Abdul Majid, Suman Fernando, Aggrey Burke, Sashi Sashidharan, John Triseliotis, Bryn David, Anni Lau, Wen-Shing Tseng, Vekoba Rao, and T. Asuni. These authors were from Africa, USA, India, Canada, and various cities in the UK known to have significant proportions of people from black and other minority ethnic groups. Their cogent, pioneering work over decades has shaped the discourse on cultural psychiatry in the UK and, even today, some of them continue to engage in constructive debates and to point out conceptual flaws in dominant models of psychiatric practice which still argue for a single curriculum and a single service into which all must fit.

Suman Fernando and Aggrey Burke have been especially courageous by speaking openly about racism and discrimination doing research, writing and publishing on the subject [2–5]. A pivotal point in the history of cultural psychiatry in the UK was almost certainly the remarkable and well-known book by Roland Littlewood and Maurice Lipsedge titled *Aliens and Alienists*, first published in 1982, and now in its third edition [6]. This volume again tackled racism but linked it with medical practice, and included discussions of depression and somatization among blacks, illness as metaphor and as communication, and the differences between normality and abnormality. The book was especially powerful as Littlewood's masterly use of ethnographic thick description made the usual nuanced academic deliberations far more accessible to students and to the public at large. The 'new cross-cultural psychiatry' movement took forward the need for a more critical and contextual understanding of mental health and mental illness. An excellent editorial by Littlewood in the *British Journal of Psychiatry* titled 'From categories to contexts: the new cross cultural psychiatry', masterfully documents these views [7]. Littlewood has been a prolific writer on topics of religion, psychiatry, and traditional and alternative systems of healing the world over. These early analyses gave way to greater interest within and outside the Royal College of Psychiatrists, with more trainees expressing interest on the subject, and more conferences emerging with themes of cultural psychiatry, cross-cultural psychiatry, transcultural psychiatry, alongside clinical studies of psychotherapy and culture. Nevertheless, there remains no dedicated curriculum for medical students or for trainee psychiatrists, most teachers and students relying on odd examination questions to motivate sufficient study; yet, there are few centres of excellence or clinical or academic institutions expressing interest and dedication to recruiting teachers, and providing high quality training and teaching on this subject.

Why We Need a Critical Cultural Psychiatry

As an enthusiastic supporter of cultural psychiatry, this artricle's author conceives it is as an essential clinical discipline and a fascinating subject for research. However, I do not see yet a coherent subject with a consistent and widely agreed definition, unique methodologies or event agreement on the most important research questions. This assertion is not new. Sashidharan made it clear in his chapter on the first edition of John Cox's book, titled '*Ideology and Politics*', and his assertions remain true today. These contradictions reflect, in part, the nature of the subject matter, a constant tension between objectivity and subjectivity, empiricism versus understanding the phenotype, the way cultures are constructed and how individuals make use (or not) of cultural factors in expressing and managing distress and dealing with life's misfortunes, as well as how they celebrate and make for positive states of mind. Clinicians want to understand their patients, but do not seem totally disposed to go beyond their primary clinical task. Internal scripts are used more and more by busy clinicians, the more experienced ones relying more on them. They seek to match what they see with what the script requires for verification or rejection of more or less stereotyped clinical hypotheses. These scripts, along with other policies and procedures, seem to be organisational and perhaps individual defences against too much emotional contact with the patient, seen as a factor that would perhaps undermine the clinical task.

Although these contradictions exist within the UK, there are reasons to suspect that they are not evident in other countries. Given that the subject of cultural psychiatry takes up one aspect of human organisation and experience, it is, however, inevitable that its practitioners are interested and active in all fields of general psychiatry. The lack of a unique identity, sets of questions, and lack of impact on policy, public health and clinical practice continue to suggest that cultural psychiatry is simply a narrative social science, practised at a distance from the realities of clinical practice. Its main challenge is whether it can produce a set of clinically relevant guidelines, and effective treatments, as well as critical and ground breaking research that improves the patient's quality of life and chances of recovery. Its main value resides not in what cultural psychiatry is but what it can achieve for all patients in multi-cultural, diverse populations as well as among people who would not be considered an ethnic minority or culturally distinct like, for example, the Irish, Welsh or Scottish in the UK.

Cultural Psychiatry in the World: A UK Perspective

Kirmayer has advanced these issues at McGill University in Montreal, with specific training programmes and a vision of the role of cultural psychiatry in future healthcare [8–10]. Thus, the role of culture in shaping experience, rather than altering its surface features is debated. The interdisciplinary training setting emphasizes the cultural history and embedding of psychiatric knowledge and practice; the social construction of ethnicity, race, and cultural identity; the impact of globalization, migration, and ideologies of citizenship on individual identity, and the configuration of cultural communities; and the integration of quantitative and qualitative ethnographic methods in basic and evaluative research. Yet, more recently, there are several new propositions about the essential nature and role of cultural psychiatry. Kirmayer writes that the field has evolved along the following lines: (1) cross-cultural comparative studies of psychiatric disorders and traditional healing, (2) efforts to respond to the mental health needs of culturally diverse populations that include indigenous peoples, immigrants, and refugees, and (3) the ethnographic study of psychiatry itself as the product of a specific cultural history. This is in sharp contrast with the early analysis of 'transcultural psychiatry' by Cox which was mostly focused on anti-racist psychiatry and power relationships [1].

The World Psychiatric Association's Transcultural Psychiatry Section (WPA-TPS) has undoubtedly been instrumental in improving communication and sharing knowledge around the world, with dedicated chairs including Wen-Shing Tseng, Ron Wintrob, Goffredo Bartocci and Rachid Bennegadi. The section was instrumental in organizing a number of symposia in WPA-sponsored meetings and events throughout the years. This active pattern was so productive that the need for cultural psychiatry and its place as a unique discipline became matters of constructive exchanges. This is an important component of the field: to invent and re-invent itself within the culture of medicine and psychiatry, within a changing society, and so also to continue to see elements of our environment, our social structures, our institutions, not as de facto natural entities but cultural constructs or products of the dominant culture in a society which may not always be friendly or receptive to the needs of cultural minorities or the less powerful to whom the term 'racialised' is being increasingly applied.

The leaders and membership of these groups worked in a dedicated and collegiate way, not fearing controversies, but, on the contrary, pushing for more space and collaboration with many other national and international associations in order to connect local realities and create a capacity for cultural psychiatry to be tested as a valuable or needed discipline around the world. This struggle resulted in the foundation of the World Association of Cultural Psychiatry (WACP), an international organisation with affiliated national associations. Its inaugural World Congress took place in Beijing, in 2006. This interconnection of local realities is essential if cultural psychiatry is to truly develop a coherent set of practices, policies, research methods and applied value in public health and social care, as well as in population well-being.

The UK Experience: Policy and Practice Experience with Delivering Race Equality

The most recent cultural product from UK health policy makers was the delivering of a race equality policy, which emerged after decades of overlooked injustices that led to poor experiences and outcomes in mental health care among minority ethnic communities, including the dramatic death of a black man in a hospital [11]. This programme had many purposes, one of which was to improve pathways to care, which had met with some successes in demonstration sites [12–14]. However, a major aim was to reduce the disproportionate representation of black people in psychiatric hospitals, as monitored by the national regulating agency carrying powers of exposure if the system did not perform in a just way. Paradoxically, with the programme in function, the disproportionate rates did not shift but became a little worse; the conclusions were that the regulator would not monitor them long enough as there was no intervention that worked, and that actually we did not understand as a society why this disproportionality existed. The policy makers wished to have nothing to do with a process that might name institutional racism as the problem [15]. At the same time, there was a need to ensure that other inequalities, based on gender, age, social exclusion, poverty, etc. were also addressed. Consequently, re-

Table 1. Examples of public mental health activities

Prevention to protect mental health, either by delaying onset or minimising disability, illness episodes, loss of social networks and financial strain
Providing models and methods to work with hard to reach groups, in order they benefit from public health interventions; this will require some targeting
Providing models and methods to work with risk behaviours and prevention: violence, self-harm, eating disorders, depression, anxiety, workplace stress, relational issues
Preventing poor health amongst those with mental health problems by encouraging take up of public health messages and interventions and specifically to minimise the health burden (beyond mental health) encountered
Preventing extreme life events with long-term mental health burden: violence, abuse
Promoting positive mental health strategies for the life course: children and learning, risk behaviours, friendships, coping with loss, understanding parental illness; elderly, working with memory and sustaining employment; for all: exercise and physical activity, nutrition, well-being and happiness, self-esteem and confidence, self-efficacy

cent policy in the UK has shifted away from an emphasis on culture or diversity or ethnicity towards public mental health and inequalities, seeking primarily for ways to prevent mental illness.

Public Health Approach and Inequalities

The strong case for a public mental health strategy exists, given the benefits to society as a whole and to those with mental health problems, in particular. This approach requires universal interventions applied to the entire population, such that the benefits are available to a greater number of people [16]. The idea is not to restrict interventions only to people who have developed an illness, and leave the rest of the population's health risks unaddressed. Effective interventions that can be used in preventive psychiatry or public mental health include preventing violence and abuse in early life, age- and gender-based violence and discrimination; creating a more balanced and empowering society in which all people from diverse age/gender/cultural backgrounds can realise their potential in work settings, whilst avoiding long periods of sickness and absence from work due to illness; providing information to the population on how to maximise their health and prevent illness, by taking lifestyle and behavioural, social, psychological and physical measures. Prevention applies generally but it could benefit especially population groups at higher risk. Many of these interventions aim to act over the life course and protect and promote what has been called 'mental capital' [17].

To some extent, mental health professionals, including psychiatrists, are already undertaking activities that have a preventive function (table 1). Ironically, cultural psychiatrists have been arguing for more indigenous systems of help and recovery, which were largely seen as peripheral. Now these are being adopted in a generic health framework, and cultural psychiatry risks being seen as too medical, and peripheral.

The public health approach does not explicitly address ethnic or cultural inequities in use of and experience with services. However, the aim of public health policy is to reduce the development of inequalities in general by ensuring illness prevention in the first place, and specifically by tackling social determinants of illness which are unequally patterned. In other words, public health approaches deal with collective and material circumstances, education, and employment inequalities. Other approaches in policy and legislation focus on stigma and discrimination in the workplace and in society in general. The risk of such an approach is that some sectors of society may be unwilling or less able to hear about these approaches, take them up or adhere to them. This might involve those with poorer educational and social status, those whose lifestyle already compromises their health and, therefore, find it hard to change their risk behaviours, those who might already suffer with severe health problems, or those who are already socially excluded to some extent and have multiple problems (i.e. homeless populations, those exposed to discrimination or stigma). These are all realities in the UK.

Patients with severe mental illness fall within this group, of course. It is even possible that such groups will fall further behind in terms of health improvements, and that the inequality gap may widen. This is not an issue confined to people with mental health problems, but has also been found in other areas of medicine, for example, cardiovascular medicine [18, 19]. Therefore, some targeted interventions are necessary for those who are less likely to benefit from a universal approach. It is possible that the emphasis on young people in such endeavours may inadvertently discriminate against older populations, so actions are needed to embrace preventive approaches among the latter.

Furthermore, not mentioning discrimination on the basis of race, ethnicity, religion and culture in current public health policies reflects, in part, the broad and overarching scope of such policies. These issues of oversight are common to various population segments such as people with learning difficulties, older populations, refugees and asylum seekers, forensic psychiatry cases, homeless populations, lesbian, gay, bisexual and transgendered groups, each of whom will require specific consideration, engagement and roll out of policies and actions that improve their health status and prevent illness.

Conclusions

When inequality issues are discussed in the UK, concerns are raised about resources, social justice, and how to tackle such matters. Regressive actions may emerge relatively easily when change is expected from providers, commissioners and policy makers. Public mental health actions at the population level should not undermine or remove actions at other levels, including that of individual practitioners. All these factors have an extraordinary impact on the development of cultural psychiatry's theory and practice. The challenges are substantial and should remain a priority in need of close attention. The good work that has gone on for decades in improving knowledge, skills and attitudes, and the evidence base for health care provision to diverse cultural groups should not be eroded or diminished. Many of the mechanisms of therapeutic failure or treatment breakdown that are discussed in other chapters in this book can also be discerned at organizational and societal levels. Thus, the British experience continues to encompass concern about ethnic and cultural inequalities in admission and detention in psychiatric hospitals, their management, understanding and improvement by means of diverse and alternative systems of care and care practices.

References

1 Cox J: Transcultural Psychiatry. Beckenham, Croom Helm, 1986.
2 Burke AW: Is racism a causatory factor in mental illness? Int J Soc Psychiatry 1984;30:1–3.
3 Burke AW: Racism and psychological disturbance among West Indians in Britain. Int J Soc Psychiatry 1984;30:50–68.
4 Fernando S: Racism as a cause of depression. Int J Soc Psychiatry 1984;30:41–49.
5 Fernando S: Studies into issues of 'race' and culture in psychiatry. Psychol Med 1998;28:496–497.
6 Littewood R, Lipsedge M: Aliens And Alienists: Ethnic Minorities and Psychiatry. London, Routledge, 1997.
7 Littlewood R: From categories to contexts: a decade of the 'new cross-cultural psychiatry'. Br J Psychiatry 1990;156:308–327.
8 Kirmayer LJ, Rousseau C, Corin E, Groleau D: Training researchers in cultural psychiatry: the McGill-CIHR Strategic Training Program. Acad Psychiatry 2008;32:320–326.
9 Kirmayer LJ, Minas H: The future of cultural psychiatry: an international perspective. Can J Psychiatry 2000;45:438–446.
10 Gold I, Kirmayer LJ: Cultural psychiatry on Wakefield's procrustean bed. World Psychiatry 2007;6:165–166.
11 Bhui K, Ascoli M, Nuamh O: The place of race and racism in cultural competence: what can we learn from the English experience about the narratives of evidence and argument? Transcult Psychiatry 2012;49:185–205.
12 Bhui K: Editorial – Enhancing pathways into care & recovery: from specialist services to healthy minds. Int Rev Psychiatry 2009;21:425–426.
13 Sass B, Moffat J, Bhui K, McKenzie K: Enhancing pathways to care for black and minority ethnic populations: a systematic review. Int Rev Psychiatry 2009;21:430–438.
14 Moffat J, Sass B, McKenzie K, Bhui K: Improving pathways into mental health care for black and ethnic minority groups: a systematic review of the grey literature. Int Rev Psychiatry 2009;21:439–449.
15 McKenzie K, Bhui K: Institutional racism in mental health care. BMJ 2007;334:649–650.
16 Rose GR: The Strategy of Preventive Medicine. Oxford, Oxford University Press, 1992.
17 Jenkins R, Meltzer H, Jones PB, et al: Foresight Mental Capital and Wellbeing Project. Mental health: future challenges. London, XXX, 2008.
18 Capewell S, Graham H: Will cardiovascular disease prevention widen health inequalities? PLoS Med 2010;7:e1000320.
19 Cooney MT, Dudina A, Whincup P, et al: Re-evaluating the Rose approach: comparative benefits of the population and high-risk preventive strategies. Eur J Cardiovasc Prev Rehabil 2009;16:541–549.

Dr. Kamaldeep Bhui
University of London, Hon Consultant Psychiatrist
East London Foundation Trust
22 Commercial Street, London E1 6LP (UK)
E-Mail k.s.bhui@qmul.ac.uk

Alarcón RD (ed): Cultural Psychiatry.
Adv Psychosom Med. Basel, Karger, 2013, vol 33, pp 40–55 (DOI: 10.1159/000348730)

Opening Up Mental Health Service Delivery to Cultural Diversity: Current Situation, Development and Examples from Three Northern European Countries

Sofie Bäärnhielm[a] · Cecilie Jávo[b] · Mike-Oliver Mösko[c]

[a]Transcultural Centre, Stockholm County Council, Stockholm, Sweden; [b]Sámi National Centre for Mental Health (SANKS), Karasjok, Norway; [c]Department of Medical Psychology, University Medical Center, Hamburg-Eppendorf, Germany

Abstract

There are inequalities in health among migrants and local populations in Europe. Due to migration, Germany, Norway and Sweden have become ethnic culturally diverse nations. There are barriers to mental health care access for refugees, migrants and minorities, and problems with quality of culturally sensitive care in the three countries. This is despite tax-funded health care systems based on equity in service provision. There is a need to develop culturally sensitive mental health services that respond to the increasing diversity of the populations. In this chapter, we will take a closer look at cultural diversity in the countries in question, discuss challenges and give examples of current work to open up mental health services to cultural diversity. The German example will focus on the movement of *Interkulturelle Öffnung* (cross-cultural opening of the health care system) and work on creating national guidelines and quality standards. From Norway, the work of the National Centre for Mental Health for the indigenous Sámi population will be presented. The Swedish example will focus on the work carried out by the Transcultural Centre. The latter is a competence centre supporting development of culturally sensitive care as an integrated part of the regional health and mental health care system in Stockholm. Finally, the relevance of mental health care for a culturally diverse population, as a part of the larger social project of building tolerant multicultural societies, will be discussed.

Migration changes European demography and challenges mental health care services [1]. In the European Union's (EU) 27 states, there are currently 47.3 million foreign-born residents, corresponding to 9.4% of the total population [2], 1.6 million recognised refugees and about 514,000 stateless people [3]. In 2004, the Council of the European Union developed a set of *Common Basic Principles on Integration* [4], among which the acceptance of diverse cultures and immigrants' right to access to health care institutions as well as to public services on a basis equal to national citizens and in a non-discriminatory way, are prominent [2]. Despite this proclamation many migrants and ethnic minorities in European countries have less access to the existing health and social services [1, 6]. Thus, a main challenge for European health care system is the provision of accessible, equitable, and good quality of care for all [7]. This includes responding to the cultural diversity of the population, to the health consequences of forced migration, to acculturation problems, and to refugee trauma, among many specific needs.

The aim of this chapter is to present current examples from three European countries working to open up mental health care services to the cultural diversity of their populations. Pertinent information regarding cultural diversity, present situation and future challenges for mental health services will be discussed.

Mental Health Care for Migrants in Europe

An increasing body of research shows inequalities in health among migrants and local populations in Europe [8]. In several European countries migration is associated with lower access to, and use of inpatient and outpatient mental health care services [9, 10]. In an overview study of prevalence of mental disorders, access and utilization of mental health and psychosocial care of migrants in Europe, Lindert et al. [6] concluded that data on migrants' mental health are scarce. Furthermore, the study showed that in many European countries migrants fall outside the existing health and socials services, especially asylum seekers and undocumented migrants. Many European countries do not have specific policies to address access to health services for migrants and ethnic minorities. Only 11 of 25 European countries had established national policies [8]. The European Commission has stated that migrants, the elderly and people with mental disorders are among the most vulnerable patient groups having significant difficulties in accessing health care services [11].

In addition to barriers in health care utilization, there are several challenges to the quality of mental health services for migrants and ethnic minorities. Health and mental professionals from 16 European countries, working in areas with a high density of migrants, pointed out eight types of problem in their health care delivery, and described components of what they considered to be good practice [7]: language barriers, difficulties due to health care coverage, social deprivation and traumatic experiences, lack of familiarity with the health care system, cultural differences, different understandings of illness and treatment, negative attitudes among staff and patients, and lack of access to medical history. As components of good practice to overcome these problems they suggested organisational flexibility, sufficient time and resources, good interpreters; services, working with families and social services, cultural awareness of staff, and clear guidelines as to the entitlements of care for the different groups.

Culture and Mental Health Services in Germany

Germany currently has 15.7 million people with a so-called migration background. According to the definition of the national micro-census these are foreign-born residents and their offspring who have immigrated to Germany since 1950. This equals 19.3% of the general population of 81.7 million. One third of people with a migration background are born in Germany. More than half of this population (55%) has German citizenship. The largest migration groups comprise people with roots in Turkey (3.0 million), in the succession states of the former Soviet Union (2.9 million) and in the succession states of the former Yugoslavia (1.5) [12].

Refugees and asylum seekers constitute another important group as Germany today is the industrialized nation with the largest refugee population reaching almost 400,000 (in 2011), and including 45,741 new asylum seekers [3]. Before significant changes in the Asylum Procedure Act, more than 433,000 new asylum seekers were registered in 1992 [13]. According to estimates, between 100,000 and 1,400,000 people without a legal residence permit currently live in Germany. Basic rights as well as social and health care standards are withheld or cannot be asserted because of fear of detection and deportation [14].

Current National Politics toward Multiculturalism

For several decades the possibilities of participating in society were limited for people without German citizenship [15]. The political will to perceive Germany as an immigration country was missing for a long time. The enacting of the immigration law in 2005 paved the way for Germany to move from being an informal to a formal immigration country [16]. The successful integration of migrants became a national priority in all societal domains such as the labour market and education. The National Integration Plan [17], the Federal Integration Summits as well as the German Islam Conference emphasize the political efforts made by Germany as an integration country.

To evaluate the political integration goals, an integration monitoring system as well as scientific reports on indicators of integration has been developed [18]. In order to make public institutions such as administration, schools and the police more accessible to migrants, a movement called *Interkulturelle Öffnung* (cross-cultural opening) has increasingly expanded. Major practical instruments of this movement are cross-cultural competence training for employees, and the recruitment of migrants as staff members.

Cross-Cultural Aspects of Mental Health Care Services in Germany

Since the 1980s the 'interkulturelle Öffnung' has been run mainly by professionals from the mental health care system. The 12 Sonnenberger Guidelines [19] were a national initiative by health professionals to improve psychiatric-psychotherapeutic health care services and primary care for migrants in Germany. The Guidelines suggested a number of quality standards such as: facilitating access to mental health care services by providing cross-cultural sensitivity and cross-culturally competent staff; using interpreters with some psychology training; providing information in migrants' native languages; offering further education in cross-cultural psychotherapy for mental health care staff, and initiating research projects in the field of mental health and migration.

Though improvements have been made in the mental health care system, e.g. by implementing culturally and linguistically specialized treatment programmes, recruiting multi-cultural staff, and implementing cross-cultural issues in the (further) training of health professionals, more remains to be achieved. The German mental health care system has not reached the level that is culturally and linguistically fully oriented to the needs of its diverse patient population, a situation that is fully documented by research findings. With regard to inpatient mental health care utilization rate of patients with a migration background a general under-supply is indiscernible, as the number of re-settlers (i.e. migrants with a German origin from the former Soviet Union) equates to its proportion in the general population. Nevertheless, the utilization rate by patients without German citizenship is up to three times lower than that of patients who are German citizens [20, 21]. In outpatient mental health care services the proportion of patients with a migration background is half compared to its proportion in the general population [10].

The cultural and linguistic diversity of outpatient mental health care professionals is limited as therapists with a migration background are underrepresented. One of the serious consequences of this reality is that patients who are not able to speak sufficient German or the common European foreign languages are practically excluded from outpatient mental health care services as the cost of interpreters is not covered by health insurance [10].

With regard to process-related cross-cultural issues, findings show a high psychopathological burden of allochthonous patients amongst those receiving inpatient treatment for mental/psychosomatic disorders when compared to German patients. The highest burden is measured for Turkish patients and patients from former Yugoslavia [20]. The outcome findings for inpatient mental health care patients show that there is no negative treatment effect for migrants in general compared to German patients. Closer examination of the different migrant groups shows that Turkish patients and patients from former Yugoslavia have the lowest treatment outcome levels [22, 20].

Relevant negative predictors for treatment outcome are clinical as well as socio-economic factors. Migration background alone, however, does not account for the significant variance [20]. Also, health care provider factors can have a negative influence on the treatment process. Encounters with 'foreign' patients on a psychiatric inpatient unit triggered negative emotions amongst staff, and had a detrimental effect upon the development of a patient-provider relationship and treatment outcome [23]. How significant the challenge in the clinical exchanges with a patient from a different cultural background can be is shown by a study of outpatient psychotherapists. Though the majority had more than 20 years of professional experience, two thirds mentioned substantial challenges in their work with patients with a migration background (e.g. divergent value system, communication and language problems, different explanatory models of disease and the healing process, lack of adherence to treatments) [10].

In the light of a growing number of culturally diverse patients, cross-cultural competence is becoming a basic requirement for (mental) health care providers. The importance of cross-cultural aspects in (further) training of (mental) health care providers is emphasized by three developments. First, 83.3% of the directors of psychiatric training institutions reported a demand for training in transcultural psychiatry [24]. Second, in the context of a nationwide initiative for the academic education of medical students' national competence-based learning, objectives for cross-cultural competence are being defined [21]. Third, nationwide quality standards in cross-cultural competence training for (prospective) psychotherapists, similar to the Canadian guidelines for training in Cultural Psychiatry, are being developed [25].

The standard mental health care service for asylum seekers is very limited in Germany due to legal restrictions. Coverage of the cost of treatment by health insurance takes place only in the presence of acute disease or pain conditions. Several non-governmental organisations (NGOs) around the country (e.g. the Centre for Torture Victims in Berlin) offer specialized social, psychological and medical treatment for refugees and surviving victims of organized crime. A standard mental health care service for people without legal residence status does not exist. Local funding initiatives have been established in a few cities in order to cover health care service expenses. NGOs mainly offer basic medical health care service by working with a network of health care providers who provide services on an honorary basis.

An Example of Delivering Culturally Sensitive Care

There are approximately two dozen clinical initiatives delivering culturally and linguistically sensitive inpatient care, mainly for Turkish-speaking patients. One example is the Rehabilitation Clinic for Psychosomatic Medicine and Psychotherapy in Bad Segeberg, which for the past 20 years has offered a specialised inpatient treatment program for these patients. Like several other clinics in Germany, specialising in the needs of particular migrant groups, a multimodal treatment concept is offered, consisting of individual and group psychotherapy, psychopharmacotherapy, psychoeducation, art and exercise therapy, relaxation training, social competence training and other services. The specialised programme for Turkish-speaking patients is offered by a team of bilingual doctors, nurses and psychotherapists. For chronic, multimorbid patient groups with lower educational level, the treatment goals as well as the treatment concepts are adjusted to their resources. Information as well as basic documentation is offered in the Turkish language [26].

Culture and Mental Health Services in Norway

The Migrants

Norway has long remained a monocultural society, except for the indigenous Sámi people in the northern parts of the country. However, in recent years, there has been a major demographic change due to migration. This change has taken place within a short period of time, leading to a 5-fold increase in foreign-born citizens in only one generation. The first migrants were workers, mainly from Pakistan, Turkey and Morocco. Later, as labour immigration from countries outside the European economic zone was banned, the majority of migrants were refugees or asylum seekers from Asia, Africa and Latin America. Asylum seekers to Norway reached its peak in 2002.

The expansion of the EU in 2004 led to a marked increase in work-seeking migrants from the new East-European member states. In 2010, work remained the major reason for immigration to Norway and 64% of the immigrants came from EU countries (i.e. Schengen member states) [27]. Although Norway is not a member of the EU, it has signed the *Schengen Agreement* which involves eliminating border controls with other Schengen member states, while simultaneously strengthening border controls with non-member states.

The number of people with a migration background is increasing. Net immigration at the beginning of 2012 was the highest ever recorded. In addition to legal migration, there has been a sharp increase in the amount of illegal migrants, the number of which remains unknown. Today, there are 655,000 first- and second-generation migrants living in Norway. They come from more than 219 different countries and self-governed regions and constitute 13.1% of the total population (of about 5 million). A rather high proportion (44%) comes from countries in Asia, Africa and South and Central America [28].

Up until now, attitudes towards migration have been rather liberal in Norway compared to other European countries. In a survey mapping the populations' political, social, moral and religious attitudes in different European countries [29], Norway ranks amongst the most migration-friendly countries, including the willingness to receive immigrants from non-Western countries. However, even in a liberal and democratic country such as Norway, racism and anti-migrant attitudes do exist, however. Due to the current economic crisis and resulting unemployment, attitudes may well become more anti-immigration.

National Minorities and the Sámi

As mentioned above, other Minority groups in Norway include Kven (Finns), the Roma and Jews. The Roma, in particular, have experienced various types of state oppression and racism in former periods [30]. Although the official policy today is different, Norway has been criticized by the Helsinki Committee for Human Rights for not doing enough to protect their language and culture and stop discrimination.

In addition, Norway has an indigenous population, the Sámi. The Sámi people inhabits the circumpolar region of Scandinavia, Finland and northwest Russia. Of a total population of 50,000–100,000, at least 70% live in Norway. Like the North American native peoples (Indians and Inuit) in Alaska and Canada, the Inuit in Greenland and the aboriginal peoples of northern Russia, they are Arctic people. Traditionally, their society was based on hunting and gathering. Until recent times, a nomadic life style was prevalent, reindeer-herding being one of their main ways of living. Today, only a smaller proportion of the population makes a living as reindeer herders. Their lifestyle, culture and language differ greatly from those of the Norwegians. Due to a long-standing history of discrimination and a forced assimilation policy by the national authorities, a large proportion of the Sámi have lost their ethnic identity and native language [31].

The aim of former Norwegian policies was to erase their identity. Hence, Sámi children were placed in Norwegian boarding schools and the Sámi language was forbidden in schools. Only those citizens who could read and write Norwegian were entitled to buy land. In the 1960s, due to a more liberal ideological climate and general ideas about human worth and the rights of small nations, this 'norwegianization' policy was altered. Forced assimilation was replaced by a process of integration, and of ethnic revival within the society itself [32].

In 1988, a new paragraph (§110a) was added to the Norwegian constitution, acknowledging the Sámi as a people, and their right to develop their own language, culture and social life. In 1990, Norway ratified the United Nation's ILO convention No. 169 on indigenous peoples, which further strengthened the rights of the Sámi. Today, the Sámi have gained their own parliament and jurisdiction area in which Sámi and Norwegian languages are granted equal status as official languages. Within this area, the Sámi population has legal right to all public services in their own language, including health services.

The Need for Mental Health Services: Current Situation
Mental health problems in the Norwegian migrant population are three times higher than in the general population [34, 35]. When different groups of migrants are compared, large intergroup differences emerge both in the prevalence of actual diseases and in risk factors. For instance, the prevalence of mental problems in migrants from middle- and low-income countries is more than twice that of migrants from high-income countries and second generation migrants.

Few cross-cultural studies have been carried out on mental health and utilization of health services in the indigenous Sámi population. In 2003–2004, a health survey was performed in the Sámi areas, showing a similar pattern of social differences in health in Sámi and Norwegian populations [35]. However, the Sámi reported more health problems than Norwegians, especially in the more assimilated areas, suggesting that ill-health might be connected with experiences of discrimination and assimilation [36]. Other studies have found that Sámi-speaking patients were less satisfied with primary health services [37], and that Sámi patients treated in a psychiatric hospital showed less treatment satisfaction [38].

Equity in Norwegian Mental Health Care: Ideals and Realities
The Norwegian public health care system is primarily based on state-funded provision with a structure geared to three levels of supply – national, regional and local. An important national goal is to ensure equity in all health care, bringing health differentials down to the lowest level possible. All Norwegian citizens, regardless of geography, socio-

economic status, functional capacity, gender, sexual orientation, religion and ethnic belonging have equal rights to public health services, both within primary and secondary care. Citizens are insured by the National Insurance Scheme, which is universal and funded by taxation on income. Hence, admission to psychiatric hospitals and clinics is free, and the same goes for outpatient psychiatric consultations, except for a small user charge.

People suffering from chronic psychiatric illness are exempt from any healthcare costs. Psychiatric services are decentralized in order to be available to all citizens and geographic regions. Organizing a country's mental health care in this way might be beneficial to all the population, including migrants and ethnic minorities. However, illegal migrants do not have the same rights to public health care as persons legally resident in Norway. There is a continuing debate concerning if and how their need for services should be met.

In spite of the equity policy, many ethnic minority patients in Norway do not enjoy equal access and equal quality of mental healthcare compared to the majority population. This is due to various kinds of barriers, especially language and cultural barriers, besides lack of proper information about available services. On the whole, Norwegian mental health care providers have little or no training in culturally sensitive communication, or in systematic cultural/contextual assessment and treatments. Moreover, there is a lack of mental health professionals with minority and migrant backgrounds. Professional interpreters are few, infrequently available, and their qualifications are not always satisfactory. Many health workers do not know how to use interpreters in a professional way [39].

Improving Service Delivery: Example of the Sámi National Centre for Mental Health
In order to improve service delivery to migrants, refugees and ethnic minorities, three national competence centres have been established by the Norwegian authorities: The Norwegian Centre for Minority Health Research (NAKMI), The Norwegian Centre for Violence and Traumatic Stress Studies (NKVTS), and The Sámi National Centre for Mental Health (SANKS).

The Sámi National Centre for Mental Health was established in 2002 and is situated on the Arctic tundra, in the northernmost county of Norway and amidst the population it is supposed to serve (www.sanks.no). It is a multi-professional training centre for Sámi mental health workers, and many of the therapists are Sámi-speaking. Unlike the other competence centres mentioned above, SANKS offers psychiatric treatment and assessment to patients in addition to counselling, teaching and research. Treatment modalities include various outpatient treatments as well as treatments at psychiatric wards for adults, youth and families. Due to the long distances between the Sámi municipalities, smaller branches have been established in some other regions, and telecommunication is frequently used.

Providing mental health services for the Sámi people by establishing a Sámi competence centre has been controversial. It was argued that the mental health system was sufficient to meet the needs of Sámi patients and that there was no need for a separate institution. Besides, some warned that creating a special service might stigmatize the Sámi. Moreover, Sámi patients might not want to use such a service within their own settlements due to transparency problems. On the other hand, Sámi politicians and many health professionals claimed that the existing mental health services were not adapted to Sámi culture, and that to ensure equity the best solution was to establish a centre in which Sámi-speaking clinicians could provide therapy in their own language and conduct research in order to develop more culturally adapted clinical services. This struggle continued for several years. Finally, the Norwegian parliament provided the financial resources needed to launch the project.

The SANKS model, with a strong base within the main Sámi settlement and smaller satellites in other areas inhabited by the Sámi, has been successful. The institution has been accepted by Sámi society, and is used by Sámi patients as well as by Norwegians [40]. It has recruited and trained many Sámi professionals in mental health, and several clinicians have gained a doctoral degree. Assessments and treatments has been culturally adapted to meet the needs of the population. Moreover, counselling and teaching are offered to other mental health institutions and also to the primary care services. In an indigenous people's mental health perspective, SANKS represents a unique type of institution.

Culture and Mental Health Services in Sweden

Migration has made Sweden a highly culturally diverse nation. Economically, Sweden is characterized by an open export-oriented economy where foreign trade constitutes 95% of the GDP [41]. Migration to Sweden has mainly taken place during the post-war periods and major changes in migration patterns have taken place over the years. Until the mid-1970s this was primarily workers' migration to fulfil rising demands for labour in an expanding industry. Later, refugees and family reunion patterned migration [42]. Refugee migration has been influenced by major conflicts in the world. Labour migration has increased over the past 10 years. In 2008, the Swedish parliament embraced new regulations for labour migration; these facilitated migration from non-EU/EES countries. Labour migration is regulated by employers' labour needs. The labour migrants come from old and new EU union countries, Poland and the Baltic states among the latter. The number of migrants from non-EU Countries has also increased [43].

The proportion of the population with a foreign-born background and a non-European background is also constantly increasing. Today, first- and second-generation migrants in Sweden constitute 18.6% [44] of the population. The main country of origin is Finland, followed by Iraq and former Yugoslavia/Serbia Montenegro. In 1999, the Swedish parliament acknowledged the existence of historical national minorities. These groups are Sámi, Finns domiciled in Sweden, Torne Valley descendants, the Roma and Jews. Approximately 15,000–20,000 Sámi people live in Sweden. Recently, Sweden was criticized by the rapporteur of the UN's Human Rights Council for the lack of a national health policy for the Sámi population and lack of a Sámi health research centre such as can be found in Norway [45].

For a long time, the point of departure for the general official Swedish integration policy has been that integration should be based on the society's ethnic and cultural diversity. The objectives of the integration policy are equal rights, responsibilities and opportunities for all, regardless of ethnic or cultural background; a community based on diversity; a society characterised by mutual respect and tolerance, in which everyone, irrespective of his or her background, can take an active and responsible part [46].

There is a discrepancy between official policy and reality. For migrants in Sweden, especially women, the level of employment has decreased year after year; the average income is lowest for people born in Africa and Asia; foreign-born women have the highest ill-health figures, and men born in Sweden the lowest, and there is also well-documented ethnic housing segregation [47].

Challenges for Cultural Psychiatry

A compelling amount of facts and research in Sweden point to unequal health care with several groups of migrants, especially refugees, being more exposed groups for somatic [48] as well as mental health problems [49]. Many groups of refugees have a background of organized violence and torture [49, 50]. Migration has been shown to be a risk factor for psychosis for several groups in Sweden [51, 52], especially for second-generation migrants [53] and black migrants from developing countries [54]. Acculturative stress has an impact on mental health. Data from an annual national survey in Sweden showed that Turkish-born immigrants in Sweden had a significantly increased risk of self-reported anxiety, sleeping problems and severe pain, even after adjusting for age and socio-economic status [55].

The Swedish health care system is funded by taxation, organized by counties and based on everyone's equal right to health care [42]. Ways of responding to cultural diversity in Swedish mental health care has shifted due to migration patterns and politics. Immigrant rights first became an issue in connection with labour migration from Finland in the 1960s [56], and the right to interpreters was introduced then. The use of interpreters free of charge still exists. In the 1980s, when groups of refugees arrived, trauma clinics were set up in several counties. The clinics have been important for traumatized patients and knowledge development. Over the years there have been several local, time-limited projects in different parts of Sweden focusing upon improving care for refugees and migrants (for a further account, see Bäärnhielm et al. [42]).

Undocumented migrants in Sweden have until now been excluded from tax-funded care, and adult asylum seekers are only offered subsidized care that cannot be deferred [57]. This is criticized both nationally and internationally. Sweden is described as one of the most restrictive EU countries in providing health care for asylum seekers [58], in contradiction to international conventions about human rights that Sweden has signed. A very active movement advocates improving care for undocumented migrants and asylum seekers, arguing that health care should be seen as a human right issue, independent of migration politics. The movement includes health professionals, medical organisations, trade unions and religious groups. In line with medical ethics and human rights, an inquiry set up by the government has suggested that 'availability of health care and the associated obligations and benefits should be based on equal conditions for those who stay within the country, regardless of whether they have the necessary permit to stay in the country or not' [57].

Improving Service Delivery – Example of the Transcultural Centre in Stockholm
With the aim of improving mental health care for the increasingly culturally diverse population in the Swedish capital, Stockholm, a Transcultural Centre was established in 1999 by the Stockholm County Council. It started as a knowledge centre for transcultural psychiatry. Cultural diversity was seen as a concern and challenge for the whole regional mental health care system, and there was a conviction that patients, regardless of cultural, religious and ethnical background, had the right to good service in the whole mental health care system. To fulfil these requirements professionals were in need of consultative support and improved knowledge. The catchment area of the Transcultural Centre encompasses services in the greater Stockholm area with a total population of 1.9 million, over one fifth of the Swedish population.

Over the years, the work scope of the Transcultural Centre has expanded and today it includes support in the following areas: transcultural psychiatry; somatic and psychiatric care for asylum seekers and newly arrived refugees childcare for asylum seekers; dental care for asylum seekers and undocumented migrants, and health information to refugees and minorities. The Transcultural Centre supports health professionals by training, supervision and consultations, networking, knowledge transference and support of local clinical developmental work. Migrants and refugees are supported by health advisors providing oral information about health, health promotion and how the health care system works.

Supporting Health and Mental Health Professionals
Knowledge transference to professionals is performed by education and training, supervision, the Centre's website, an electronic free of charge newsletter, and training materials, and networking with several established networks of professionals. The Centre organises several training activities for health and mental health professionals with diverse professional affiliations. Among other things, it has established training programmes, including a 1-week advanced course in transcultural psychiatry. For more than 10 years this course was organised in affiliation with McGill University in

Canada. At local work places, the Centre organises tailor-made training programmes based on needs-led assessments among the staff [59]. Local training sessions on specific topics are also arranged.

The Centre offers professionals in Stockholm consultative support in their clinical work. Staff of all professional categories in the whole region can contact the centre with questions related to patients and clinical issues free of charge. Staff from the Centre can arrange in-house services and visit clinical settings for supervision and consultations. For distant institutions, video conferences are used. Consultation and supervision give an opportunity to promote multidisciplinary reflectiveness and to relate clinical cases to theoretical knowledge. Many of the consultation questions are related to difficulties in decoding a patient's language of distress, and categorizing symptoms into the diagnostic labels of ICD and DSM. Treatment difficulties and compliance in cross-cultural situations are also often addressed.

The Centre has worked to introduce the Outline for a Cultural Formulation (CF) of DSM-IV [60] into mental health care in Stockholm as it offers an interesting approach for understanding culture and context on an individualized, non-stereotyping basis. To facilitate clinical use, an interview guide for using the CF has been written in Swedish [61], clinical research on its application has been carried out [62, 63], and courses and local clinical training focusing upon using the CF have been organised. The CF is now included in the shared IT system for medical records all over Stockholm and in the regional guidelines for diagnosis and treatment of anxiety disorders.

Supporting Refugees and Immigrants

Until recently, little was done in Sweden to inform newly arrived refugees and immigrants about health, health-promoting strategies and how the health and mental health care system works. Over the past years projects with health advisors have been established in some counties in Sweden. In Stockholm, the work with health advisors started as a project funded by the EU Refugee Fund and is now part of the regular work of the Transcultural Centre.

The health advisors work with groups of refugees and immigrants in their native languages and in dialogue form, discussing migration, acculturative stress, health, health-promoting strategies and informing about how the health care system works. The health advisors meet with the groups in the local municipalities up to twelve times and get to know a great deal about the situation in the immigrant and refugee groups. This knowledge can be conveyed to health and mental health professionals via the Centre's training and consultation activities. The health advisors strive to familiarise refugees and migrants with the health and mental health care system. Further, building bridges between minority groups and health professionals has the potential of changing negative attitudes among both staff and patients.

Discussion

The European Union and other European countries have the ambition of accepting diverse cultures and stress immigrants' rights to have access to mental health care in an equal and non-discriminatory way. Despite this basic principle, there are problems concerning care of migrants, refugees and ethnic minorities. Like other European countries, Germany, Norway and Sweden face several challenges in developing and adapting mental health services to the needs of a rapidly increasing, multicultural population. In all three countries, some efforts have been made to provide culturally sensitive mental health services. Further development depends on national and regional political attitudes towards multiculturalism, migration and refugee reception as well as on the organisation of the health and mental health care services.

In Germany, medical education, research and health care services are increasingly becoming the focus of attention. The development of quality standards, the implementation of culturally and linguistically sensitive care and cross-cultural training elements in health care education are parts of the movement *Interkulturelle Öffnung*. In Norway, three national competence centres have been established: one for minority research, one for traumatic stress studies and one for mental health services for the indigenous Sámi population. In the latter, research is combined with mental health care delivery for the Sámi community. Sweden has had clinical centres for trauma victims since the 1980s and interpreters are free of charge. In Stockholm, Sweden, a transcultural competence centre has been established to support the development of culturally sensitive care as an integrated part of the regional health and mental health care system. In all three countries there are movements to advocate improved access to, and funding of, care and mental health care for asylum seekers and undocumented migrants.

A major force in the process of opening up mental health care delivery to respond to the needs of refugees, migrants and ethnic minorities in Sweden, Norway and Germany, are health and mental health professionals. In the long run, development of culturally-sensitive care requires institutionalized support, long-term funding, research, guidelines and quality standards including concerns for culture, education of students and training of staff. To turn a mental health system based on an ethnocentric perspective towards cultural diversity is a long-term project. A key element in developing culturally-sensitive care is the elaboration of clinical models that address culture in ways that are helpful and meaningful for both patients and clinicians. Instruments like the Cultural Formulation in DSM-5 are promising for taking cultural context into account in psychiatric diagnosing. Another important factor in improving culturally-sensitive care is consumer participation where individuals and minority groups can influence and guide treatments that are in tune with culturally based needs.

Conclusion

Access to good mental health care should be the right of every individual. On a national level, it is part of the larger project of building a tolerant multicultural society. In an essay on multicultural medicine, Kirmayer [64] argues that intercultural health care may contribute to the larger project of building a pluralistic society that allows the co-existence and co-evolution of diverse human traditions. He points out that the clinical encounter between the patients and health professionals offers a space for exploring ways of living and working with cultural differences, a process that can promote trust by encouraging others to consider new perspectives. Such seems to be the case in the three countries examined here: although following somewhat different agendas and strategies, and moving at slightly different rhythms, an effort to understand cultural diversity and its many clinical layers appears to be a common thread in all these efforts.

References

1 Giovanni Carta M, Bernal M, Hardoy MC, Haro-Abad JM, 'Report on Mental Health in Europe' Working Group: Migration and mental health in Europe (the state of the mental health in Europe working group: appendix I). Clin Pract Epidemiol Ment Health 2005;1:13.

2 Eurostat: Population and social conditions. Statistics in focus 2011;34 http://epp.eurostat.ec.europa.eu/cache/ITY_OFFPUB/KS-SF-11–034/EN/KS-SF-11-034-EN.PDF.

3 UNHCR: UNHCR Global Trends, 2010 http://www.unhcr.org/4dfa11499.html.

4 Council of the European Union. Immigration Integration Policy in the European Union – press release. Council Document 14615/04, 2004.

5 EU: Press release, 2,618th Council Meeting, Justice of Home Affairs, Brussel, 2004.

6 Lindert J, Schouler-Ocak M, Heinz A Priebe S: Mental health, health care utilisation of migrants in Europe. Eur Psychiatry 2008;23:14–20.

7 Priebe S, Sandhu S, Dias S, Gaddini A, Greacen T, Ioannidis E, Kluge U, Krasnik A, Lamkaddem M, Lorant V, Puigpinósi Riera R, Sarvary A, Soares JJF, Stankunas M, Strassmayr C, Wahlbeck K, Welbe M, Bogic M: Good practice in health care for migrants: views and experiences of care professionals in 16 European countries. BMC Publ Health 2011;11:3–12.

8 Mladovsky P, Rechel B, Ingleby D, McKee M: Responding to diversity: an exploratory study of migrants health policies in Europe. Health Policy 2012: 105:1–9.

9 Mösko M, Pradel S, Schulz H: The care of people with a migration background in psychosomatic rehabilitation. Bundesgesundheitsbl Gesundheitsforsch Gesundheitsschutz 2011;54:465–474.

10 Mösko M, Gil-Martinez F, Schulz H: Cross-cultural opening in German outpatient mental health care service: explorative study of structural and procedural aspects. J Clin Psychol Psychother 2012:DOI: 10.1002/cpp.1785.

11 Huber M, Stanciole A, Wahlbeck K, Tamsma N, Torres F, Jelfs E, Bremne J: Quality in and equality of access to healthcare services. European Commission, 2008. http://www.ehma.org/files/HealthQuest_en.pdf.

12 Statistisches Bundesamt: Bevölkerung und Erwerbstätigkeit. Bevölkerung mit Migrationshintergrund – Ergebnisse des Mikrozensus 2010. Wiesbaden, Statistisches Bundesamt, 2011, Fachserie 1, Reihe 2.2.

13 BAMF – Bundesamt für Migration und Flüchtlinge: Das Bundesamt in Zahlen 2010. Asyl, Migration, ausländische Bevölkerung und Integration. Nürnberg, 2011.

14 Vogel D: Update report Germany. Estimate of irregular foreign residents in Germany (2010). Database on Irregular Migration, update report 2012. http://irregular-migration.net, accessed April 4, 2013.

15 Haug T: Politische Partizipation von Inländern ohne deutsche Staatsangehörigkeit in Deutschland – Ein Beitrag zu Integration und Demokratisierung? München, GRIN Verlag, 2008.

16 Bade K: Analyse: Zuwanderung und Integration in Deutschland. Magazin-Deutschland.de, 2008. http://www.magazin-deutschland.de/de/artikel/artikelansicht/article/analyse-zuwanderung-und-integration-in-deutschland.html [accessed May 7, 2012].

17 Bundesregierung: Der Nationale Integrationsplan Neue Wege – Neue Chancen. Berlin, 2007. http://www.bundesregierung.de/Content/DE/Publikation/IB/nationaler-integrationsplan.pdf?__blob=publicationFile&v=3 [accessed May 7, 2012].

18 Institut für Sozialforschung und Gesellschaftspolitik und Wissenschaftszentrum Berlin für Sozialforschung: Zweiter Integrationsindikatorenbericht. Erstellt für die Beauftragte der Bundesregierung für Migration, Flüchtlinge und Integration. 2011.

19 Machleidt W: Die 12. Sonnenberger Leitlinien zur psychiatrisch-psychotherapeutischen Versorgung von Migrantinnen in Deutschland. Nervenarzt 2002; 73:1208–1212.

20 Mösko M: Stand der psychotherapeutischen Versorgung von Frauen und Männern mit Migrationshintergrund in Deutschland. Fachtagung – AG Gender und Depression im Bündnis gegen Depression, Hannover, 2011.

21 Brzoska P, Voigtländer S, Spallek J, Razum O: Utilization and effectiveness of medical rehabilitation in foreign nationals residing in Germany. Eur J Epidemiol 2010;25:651–660.

22 Maier C: Migration und rehabilitative Versorgung in Deutschland: Ein Vergleich der Inanspruchnahme von Leistungen der medizinischen Rehabilitation und eines Indikators für Rehabilitationserfolg zwischen Rehabilitanden türkischer und nicht-türkischer Abstammung. Universität Bielefeld, 2008. http://www.uni-bielefeld.de/gesundhw/zfv/maier.pdf.

23 Wohlfart E, Hodzic S, Özbek T: Transkulturelles Denken und transkulturelle Praxis in der Psychiatrie und Psychotherapie; in Wohlfart E, Zaumseil M (Hrsg): Transkulturelle Psychiatrie – interkulturelle Psychotherapie. Springer, Berlin, 2006, pp 144–166.

24 Calliess IT, Ziegenbein M, Gosman L, Schmauss M, Berger M, Machleidt W: Intercultural competence in the psychiatric training curriculum in Germany: results of a survey. GMS Z Med Ausbild 2008;25:Doc 92.

25 Kirmayer LJ, Fung K, Rousseau C, Lo HT, Menzies P, Guzder J, Ganesan S, Andermann L, McKenzie K: Guidelines for Training in Cultural Psychiatry – position paper. Can J Psychiatry 2012;3:1–17.

26 Schmeling-Kludas C, Fröschlin R, Boll-Klatt A: Inpatient psychosomatic rehabilitation for Turkish migrants: what can be realized, what are the effects? Rehabilitation 2003;42:363–370.

27 Thorud E: International migration 2010–2011. SOPEMI report for Norway, Report 06.01.12. Oslo, Department of Migration, Ministry of Justice and the Police, 2012.

28 Statistics Norway, 2012. http://www.ssb.no/innvandring/.

29 Blom S: Comparison of attitudes in Norway and other European countries; in Henriksen K, Østby L, Ellingsen D (eds): Immigration and immigrants 2010. Oslo, Statistics Norway, 2010, pp149–158.

30 Hvinden B: Romanifolket og det norske samfunnet: følgene av hundre års politikk for en nasjonal minoritet. (The Roma and Norwegian society: consequences of a hundred years' policy for a national minority). Bergen, Fagbokforlaget, 2000.

31 Solbakk JT: The Sámi People: A Handbook. Karasjok, Davvi Girji OS, 2006.

32 Stordahl V: Identity and Saminess: expressing world view and nation. Diedut 1994;1/94:57–62.

33 Blom S: Immigrant health 2005/2006. Oslo, Statistics Norway, 2008, report 2008/35.

34 Kumar BN, Grøtvedt L, Meyer HE, Søgaard AJ, Strand BH: The Oslo Immigrant Health Profile. Oslo, The Norwegian Institute of Public Health, 2008, rapport 2008:7.

35 Næss Ø, Rognerud M, Strand BH: Sosial ulikhet i helse. En faktarapport. (Social inequality in health. A report). Oslo, Norwegian Institute of Public Health, 2007, report 2007:1.

36 Hansen KL: Ethnicity, self-reported health, discrimination and socio-economic status: a study of Sami and non-Sami Norwegian populations. Int J Circumpolar Health 2010;69:111–128.

37 Nystad T, Melhus M, Lund E: Samisktalende er mindre fornøyd med legetjenestene. (Sámi-speaking patients are less satisfied with medical services). Tidsskr Norske Lægefor 2006;126:738–740.

38 Sørlie T, Nergård JI: Treatment satisfaction and recovery in Saami and Norwegian patients following psychiatric hospital treatment: a comparative study. Transcult Psychiatry 2005;42:295–316.

39 Kale E, Kumar BN: Challenges in healthcare in multiethnic societies: Communication as a barrier to achieving health equity; in Maddock J (ed): Public Health – Social and Behavioral Health. Open Access Book, 2012, pp 295–308.

40 'Samhandlingsreformen' Govermental Report No. 47 (2008–2009). Oslo, Ministry of Health and Care Services, 2009.

41 Hatzigeorgiou A, Lodefalk M: Trade and Migration. Firm-Level Evidence, www.oru.se, 2011.

42 Bäärnhielm S, Ekblad S, Ekberg J, Ginsburg BE: Historical reflections on mental health care in Sweden. The Welfare State and cultural diversity. Transcult Psychiatry 2005;42:394–319.

43 Migrationsverket, 2:2010. Papport. Migration 200–2010. http://www.migrationsverket.se/download/18.78fcf371269cd4cda980004557/migration_sv.pdf.

44 Statistic Sweden: Statistical Yearbook of Sweden, 2011. Örebro, SCB, 2011.

45 Hunt P: Mission to Sweden. Report of the Special Rapporteur on the right of everyone to enjoyment of the highest attainable standard of physical mental health. The United Nations General Assembly. Human Rights Council, 2007, report NoA/HRC/4/28/ Add.

46 Ministry of Industry: Swedish integration policy for the 21st century, 2002. www.naring.regeringen.se.

47 Swedish Integration Board: Pocket Facts – Statistics on Integration. Stockholm, The Swedish Integration Board, 2006.

48 Hollander AC, Bruce D, Ekberg J, Burström B, Borell C, Ekblad S: Longitudinal study of mortality among refugees in Sweden. Int J Epidemiology 2012:1–9.

49 SOU, Swedish Board of Health and Social Welfare. Folhälsorapport, 2009.

50 Søndergaard HP: Post-traumatic stress disorder and life events among recently resettled refugees; diss, Stockholm, Department of Public Health Sciences, Division of Psychosocial Factors and Health, Karolinska Institutet, 2002.

51 Hjern A, Wicks S, Dalman C: Social adversity contributes to high morbidity in psychosis in immigrants – a national cohort study in two generations of Swedish residents. Psychol Med 2004;34:1025–1033.

52 Zolkowska K, Cantor-Graae E, McNeil TF: Increased rates of psychosis among immigrants to Sweden: is migration a risk factor for psychosis? Psychol Med 2001;31:669–678.

53 Leão ST, Sundquist J, Frank G, Johansson LM, Johansson SE, Sundquist K: Incidence of schizophrenia or other psychoses in first- and second-generation immigrants. A national cohort study. J Nerv Ment Dis 2006;194:27–33.

54 Cantor-Graae E, Zolkowska K, McNeil F: Increased risk of psychotic disorder among immigrants in Malmö: a 3-year first-contact study. Psychol Med 2005;35:1155–1163.

55 Steiner KH, Johansson SE, Sundquist J, Wändell PE: Self-reported anxiety, sleeping problems and pain among Turkish-born immigrants in Sweden. J Ethnicity Health 2007;12:363–379.

56 SOU 1989: 111: Underlag till Storstadsutredningen – Invandrare i Storstad (in Swedish). 1989.

57 SOU 2011: 48 Vård efter behov och på lika villkor – en mänsklig rättighet. Betänkande av Utredningen om vård för papperslösa m.fl. Elanders Sverige AB (in Swedish with a summary in English). Stockholm, 2011.

58 Norredam A, Mygind A, Krasnik A: Access to health care for asylum seekers in the European Union – a comparative study of country polices. Eur J Public Health 2006;16:286–290.

59 Bäärnhielm S, Mösko M: Cross-cultural training in mental health care – challenges and experiences from Sweden and Germany. Eur Psychiatry 27/special issue 2012:1/51–56.

60 American Psychiatric Association: Diagnostic and Statistical Manual of Mental Disorder, ed 4, text revision. Washington, American Psychiatric Association, 2003.

61 Bäärnhielm S, Scarpinati Rosso M, Pattyi L: Kultur, kontext och psykiatrisk diagnostik. Manual för intervju enligt kulturformuleringen i DSM-IV. Stockholm, Transkulturellt Centrum, Stockholms läns landsting, 2007.

62 Bäärnhielm S, Scarpinati R: The cultural formulation: a model to combine nosology and patients' life context in psychiatric diagnostic practice. Transcult Psychiatry 2009;46:406–428.

63 Scarpinati Rosso M, Bäärnhielm S: Use of the Cultural Formulation in Stockholm: a qualitative study of mental illness experience among migrants. Transcult Psychiatry 2012;49:283–301.

64 Kirmayer LJ: Multicultural medicine and the politics of recognition. J Med Philos 20110;0:1–14. http://jmp.oxfordjournals.org/content/early/2011/07/29/jmp.jhr024.short?rss=1.

Sofie Bäärnhielm, MD, PhD
Transcultural Centre, Stockholm County Council
St Göran's Hospital, Floor 13
SE–112 81 Stockholm (Sweden)
E-Mail sofie.baarnhielm@sll.se

Alarcón RD (ed): Cultural Psychiatry.
Adv Psychosom Med. Basel, Karger, 2013, vol 33, pp 56–63 (DOI: 10.1159/000348733)

Cultural Psychiatry in the French-Speaking World

Joseph Westermeyer

Department of Psychiatry, University of Minnesota, Mental Health Service, Minneapolis VA Medical Center, Minneapolis, Minn., USA

Abstract

For the last five centuries, France's international influence has been constant. This has been particularly evident in the areas of general culture, history and science. In psychiatry, the role of Pinel during the French Revolution, and the discovery of the first psychotropic agent, chlorpromazine, by Delay and Deniker are two outstanding historical facts. This chapter examines the contributions of French social scientists in the understanding of the sequelae of colonial exploitation, racism and political oppression. The establishment of a multi-ethnic society in France and Francophile regions of the world has led to the gradual creation of a cultural psychiatry rich in terminological influences, clinical understanding, training programs and research. Closer connections between French psychiatric thought and Anglophile psychiatry is likely to produce beneficial effects.

Historical Account

The sun never sets on Francophile soil. Several countries of northern, eastern, and western Africa have been strongly influenced by French psychiatry. In the Middle East, Lebanon has long had strong ties to France. The Indochinese countries of Vietnam, Cambodia, and Laos have continued their professional and medical contacts to French medicine and psychiatry. Tahiti and the nearby Pacific islands lie within the French sphere. In Haiti, French Guinea, and other Caribbean entities, both 'high French' and locally spoken French patois co-exist. Further north, in Canada, the large Quebec province speaks French as its primary language.

French international influence began with the age of discovery (from the Eurocentric perspective) in the 16th century and continued through imperial expansions in the 19th century. In some instances, French remains the predominant and legal language. In other countries, especially those whose people speak a polyglot of distinct languages, French is a common lingua franca (shared language). In these settings, French may be a market language, a language of instruction and learning, and/or an official language of the government. English is only beginning to challenge the predominance of French in some of these countries and regions, such as Indochina.

Early on, French physicians working in these distant lands brought in French diagnostic and treatment practices. Over time, thousands of people from these areas went to France for medical and later psychiatric training. Eventually, they built clinics and hospitals reflecting French style and organization, as well as practice. Thus, French psychiatric thought and practice exist around the globe at different levels of depth and expansion.

Evolution of French Psychiatry

Beginning a few centuries ago, French psychiatry yielded many innovations. These advances were first felt in France, then in its regions of influence, and finally arrived in every corner of the non-Francophile world. Perhaps the first of these modern approaches was the application of humanistic care practices toward severely mentally persons. The most notable of these changes was the striking of irons by Philippe Pinel at Hôpital Pitié-Saltpêtrière, in the midst of the French Revolution [1]. This single event heralded scores of other changes in the practice and attitude toward mentally ill people.

Later in the 19th century, French advances in psychiatric thought and practice attracted physicians from across Europe to France. Jean-Martin Charcot, later director of Pitié-Saltpêtrière, established the practice of careful description of psychopathology as well as neurological conditions [2]. He also fostered interest in treatment. His work on hypnosis enticed Sigmund Freud to study in Paris. Early interest in psychopathology was reflected in the many French names still appended to various psychiatric syndromes (e.g. Cotard or nihilistic delusions, Capgras or *illusion des sosies*, Briquet or hysteria). French curiosity extended to social factors engendering psychopathology, revealed in the syndromes *folie à deux, à famille,* and *à milieu* (madness of two, of the family, and of the group/setting). They also focused on early or pathognomonic symptoms of mental disorder that might be useful for diagnosis, treatment or prognosis, as exemplified by the symptoms *belle indifférence, déjà vu, déjà pensé, écho de pense, idée de pense,* and *mania à potu.*

Following World War II, French pharmacologists turned their attentions to psychotropic agents that might affect awareness, perceptions and mood, as well as physiological effects such as temperature and hypotension. This work had its origins in shock associated with trauma – a major interest of French military and trauma surgeons following two world wars in which France was a major participant. Early in their

Vietnam war (late 1940s and early 1950s), they employed a combination of phenergan (an antihistamine) and an opiate or opioid medication in the wounded, facilitating analgesia, alleviating fear, and opposing shock[1]. While working on similar compounds, Delay and Deniker developed the first antipsychotic agent, chlorpromazine (Largactil in French parlance, Thorazine in most Anglophile settings) at the Rhone-Poulenc Pharmaceutical Company, under the direction of Paul Charpentier (1952) [3, 4]. First studied by a French military surgeon for trauma, psychiatrists soon adapted it for its 'tranquilizing' effects.

French interest in the mind, including psychiatric disorder, invited contributions from other fields. For example, Emile Durkheim – widely considered the first sociologist – chose suicide as his topic of study [5]. Familial and societal contributions to psychopathology, as well as ameliorating influences, have received perhaps more attention in French journals than in Anglophile journals. As one of the first countries to experience a burgeoning elderly population (beginning over a century ago), the French have developed new approaches to understanding and responding humanely to geriatric illness. The same may be said of their emphasis on mental health for children, not just those presenting to emergency rooms and clinicians, but to youth at large. French psychiatry has often more readily adopted addiction services and psychopharmacology (e.g. methadone and buprenorphine maintenance) than other countries of Europe. As psychoanalysis was waning in North American, it waxed in France.

French psychiatry has linked sociopolitical themes to psychiatry more readily than occurs in Anglophile settings. An example is Frantz Fanon, born in Martinique, educated in France, and later director of an Algerian psychiatric hospital. His book, *Wretched of the Earth*, became a primer for understanding the psychological repercussions of colonial exploitation and the dehumanizing effects of racism [6]. In addition to exporting its ideas to society at large, French psychiatry has been subject to political criticism on various occasions. A recent 2008 example was the blame President Nicolas Sarkozy put on French psychiatry for the fatal stabbing of a student by a mentally ill man. Although stung by this public criticism, French psychiatry responded in such a way as to protect both patients and society insofar as feasible, as opposed to silently conforming to official sanctions or passively ignoring political criticisms.

Contributions of Social Scientists to French Cultural Psychiatry

Durkheim's work on suicide, extended to traditional cultures overwhelmed by European technology and worldviews, encompassed the concept of *anomie*, 'absence of norms' or loss of identity. A key theory of this condition describes the breakdown of

---

[1] During 1965–1967, I learned this beneficial combination from a French-trained Laotian physician with whom I worked in rural Laos.

social bonds between the individual and the community. In this perspective, *anomie* leads to moral deregulation and the disappearance of legitimate aspirations. Accepted social standards and values become meaningless. Perhaps more than other modern mega-nations, France fosters and respects its culture as a key feature in the public's optimal mental health.

The *anomie* concept has been applied to scores of aboriginal cultures that have devolved into drunkenness, violence, abuse of woman and children, anarchy, and a near-total break with their cultural past. It has also been applied to large urban populations in which many youth are marginalized and unable to achieve valued social roles or lifestyles in highly competitive, overly structured, or narrowly conceived rigid cultures. And it has been seen as the inevitable penalty that a society pays for ignoring its artists, writers, and other creative thinkers. Albert Camus, the Nobel laureate author of French-Spanish-Algerian background, addressed the personal consequences of *anomie* in his books, some of which have autobiographical overtones [7].

The role of French anthropologists has not brought them readily into collaboration with French physicians, including psychiatrists, even though in academic departments, they work in collaboration with those from other fields, such as philosophy or sociology. Anthropology researchers work in government-sponsored centers where they conduct studies relevant to ethnic groups of interest to France, such as tribal groups in former French colonies [8].

Claude Levi-Strauss greatly influenced the development of French anthropology following World War II. His contributions to the field focused on structural elements of societies. Perhaps his best known work involved kinship structures, and their reflection in linguistics. Later, he studied myths and their influence on religious beliefs and worldview perspectives [9, 10]. His seminal efforts guided the subsequent work of other anthropologists for decades. A result of this emphasis can be seen in the French psychiatric and psychological devotion to family studies.

A Multi-Ethnic Society

Until a few centuries ago, France strove for cultural homogeneity. A single religion was legal. The French language was regulated. Power flowed from the center to the periphery. Intermarriage to other nationalities was for the nobility. Courts applied constitutional rather than common law. Rather than divide government, commercial, and academic interests among several cities, Paris dominated all sectors. Although these characteristics have not totally left the scene, several factors have limited or reduced them.

One factor has been the continuity of ethnic groups within France that, while conforming for centuries, have gloried recently in their individuality. Celtic-Scandinavian groups in Normandy and other ethnic groups on borders with Belgium, Germany, Switzerland, Italy and Spain have celebrated their ethnic preferences in food and dress, sometimes even in language. Marriage to other nationalities no longer carries the opprobrium it once possessed. Religious belief, if even present, no longer divides people and communities as it once did.

Perhaps the most notable factor has been the immigration of people from colonial countries to France. Some of this migration began long ago and has continued gradually. Solis, a marketing company, estimated in 2009 that the population of France included first- and second-generation immigrants from different regions as follows: 3.3 million (5.2% of the population) from North Africa and the Middle East, 1.1 million (1.8%) sub-Saharan Africans, and 0.7 million (1.1%) people from the West Indies. People from other countries of Europe compose an even greater proportion of the population. The number of foreign-born persons in France today is estimated at about 19%, or close to that of the United States. In 2010, 27.3% of newborns in France had at least one foreign-born parent. As in the US, international adoption has also widened the French gene pool [11].

Some of these groups have formed into large ethnic enclaves where one might spend an entire day, indeed an entire lifetime steeped in the language, cuisine, and dress from the country-of-origin. This has especially been the case for people from North Africa and the Middle East. Predictably, these enclaves have sometimes descended into violence and political unrest due to poverty and to youth's inability to achieve economic equality.

Contributions of French Psychiatrists to Cultural Psychiatry

Early French interests in exploration, noted above, led to curiosity regarding the life ways and worldviews of other peoples. Early post-1500 AD missionaries and minor nobles settled into these cultures, observing, writing about them, and collecting their artifacts. These early writings include some early descriptions of abnormal or troublesome behaviors, as well as values and customs markedly different from those existent in France at the time. Intermarriage with local peoples not only deepened the understanding and appreciation of these cultures, but also facilitated syncretic evolutions of new cultural forms and practices wedding many indigenous and French traditions.

In the 1800s and later, these early adventurists gave way to later commercial domination and political colonization. Clinicians often accompanied these missions, providing services to indigenous peoples as well as the expatriate Frenchmen. Ultimately, the French established psychiatric clinics and hospitals in their colonies [12].

As one might expect, French psychiatrists brought to their colonies the French penchant for careful psychiatric description. Out of this experience arose 'foreign' syndromes that informed the burgeoning field of cultural psychiatry. One example is *bouffée délirante*, a short-lived but florid psychosis resolving within weeks, often observed in the cultures visited or occupied by the French [13]. First described by Magnon in the 1880s, it could occur with tropical infectious disease, especially those accompanied by fever or encephalitis. A psychogenic form could produce hysterical reactions, or responses to severe stress or loss. Sometimes even local versions were discerned, such as *bouffée délirante Haïti*.

Folk metaphors from Francophile countries have made their way into French expressions. Some pithy phrases have spread internationally. One phrase from Haiti, *lute sans victoire* or 'struggle without victory' depicts a bleak, meaningless life. Another phrase *soulegement par Dieu* or 'relief through God' involves finding meaning for or relief from suffering through a deity or religious practice.

Contributions to cultural psychiatry have also arisen from Francophile areas outside of France. Perhaps the most fertile source has been Canada [14], a country with both strong Francophile and Anglophile roots. This area gave rise to the journal *Transcultural Psychiatry* (earlier titled *Transcultural Psychiatric Research Reviews*). Immigrant psychiatrists from Eastern Europe, Latin America, and Asia led these initial efforts, which have been further developed by native-born Canadians of many ethnic origins.

Links in Psychiatric Thought between France and North America

Although France greatly influenced American psychiatry thought, practice, and innovation for 150 years, its influence over the last half-century has waned. Several psychiatric observers have framed the divergence as due to a collage of factors, ranging from basic worldview to historical coincidence [15–18]. Philosophical viewpoints evident in French psychiatric publications have included metaphysical matters, such as existentialism and structuralism. Meanwhile Anglophile psychiatry has valued more empirical and pragmatic approaches. French psychiatric treatises have often been rich in their linguistic metaphors, but thin in regard to hypotheses that might be scientifically tested.

The French stress on maintaining a certain independence of thought has led to innovations that would be unlikely in the Anglophile world. An example is the recent development in clinical psychosomatics. Interdisciplinary studies in French psychosomatics over the last few decades have joined several sub-fields: psychoanalysis, neuroscience, medicine, and psychotherapy. Several years ago, a 1-year training course began at Pitié-Saltpêtrière. Trainees have consisted of internists, psychiatrists, therapists, and analysts [19]. The 19 faculty members likewise reflect a range of clinical interests. This program presents a unique, yet sensible approach. It also mirrors special characteristics of the French system. Non-psychiatric academics and government funders could readily perceive the reasonableness of approaching psychosomatic problems from a diversity of fields. In most Anglophile academic and training settings, the conflicts within psychiatry would make it most unlikely that a department chair or NIH bureau chief could overcome his or her banal interests in the service of exposing trainees to many viewpoints within one field of study.

Over the years, French attitudes toward Anglophile psychiatry have perhaps been more open than the reverse in several areas. For example, French military psychiatrists remained abreast of Veterans Administration progress through regular visits of a VA psychiatrist (John Kluznik) to France. French psychiatrists collaborated with a leading American psychiatry (John Talbott) to produce a French-American psychiatric meeting on refugee mental health and other elements of social psychiatry [20]. Every year, scores of Francophile psychiatrists from around the world attend the annual meeting of the American Psychiatric Association.

Growing Anglophile interest in French psychiatry suggests a rapprochement. This movement has taken a few different forms. One example consists of growing American interest in French notions of psychopathology, such as the spectrum of mood disorder, drawn from earlier French works [21]. Another example is the energy demonstrated by the North American-based Association for the Advancement of Philosophy and Psychiatry, established in 1989. Its members reside primarily in the United States, but they also come from several other Anglophile (Britain, South Africa, Canada) and non-Anglophile countries (Italy, Netherlands, France, Japan) as well. They are devoted to the understanding of inherent links between psychiatry and various fields within philosophy.

References

1 Zilboorg G: A History of Medical Psychology. New York, Norton, 1941.
2 Owen ARG: Hysteria, Hypnosis and Healing: The Work of JM Charcot. New York, Garrett Publications, 1971.
3 Delay J, Deniker P: Le traitement des psychoses par une méthode neurolytique dérivée de l'hibernothérapie. CR Congres Med Alien Neurol France 1952;50: 497–501.
4 Thuillier J: Ten Years that Changed the Face of Mental Illness. London, Martin Dunitz, 1999.
5 Durkheim E: Le Suicide. Paris, Les Presses Universitaires de France, 1987.
6 Fanon F: Les Damnes de la Terre. Paris, 1961.
7 Todd O: Albert Camus. A Life. New York, Carroll & Graff Publishers, 2000.
8 Lemoine J: Un Village Hmong Vert du Haut Laos. Paris, Centre National de la Recherche Scientifique, 1972.
9 Levi-Strauss C: Anthropologie Structurale. Paris, Plon, 1958.
10 Levi-Strauss C: La pensée sauvage. Paris: Plon, 1962.
11 Harf A, Taieb O, et al: Externalizing behaviour problems of internationally adopted adolescents: a review (in French). Encéphale 2007;33:270–276.
12 Westermeyer J: Psychiatry in Indochina: cultural issues during the period 1965–75. Transcult Psychiatry 1977;15:23–28.
13 Pichot P: The concept of 'Bouffée délirante' with special reference to the Scandinavian concept of reactive psychosis. Psychopathology 1986;19:35–43.
14 Prince R: Transcultural psychiatry: Personal experiences and Canadian perspectives. Can J Psychiatry 2000;45:431–437.
15 Kroll J: Philosophical foundations of French and US nosology. Am J Psychiatry 1979;136:1135–1138.
16 Pichot P: Status of diagnosis and classification in the 1980's: France and the French-speaking tradition. Acta Psychiatr Belg 1983;83:115–134.

17 Dowbiggen L: Back to the future: Valentin Magnan, French psychiatry, and the classification of mental illness. Soc History Med 1996;9:383–408.

18 D'Onofrio BM, Van Hulle CA, et al: Smoking during pregnancy and offspring externalizing problems: an exploration of genetic and environmental confounds. Dev Psychopathol 2008;20:139–164.

19 Stora JB: The French group of psychoanalysis, medicine and psychosomatics: New Psychosomatics Horizons. Neuropsychoanalysis 2005;7:115–116.

20 Richetta P, Kouchner G (eds): Psychiatrie et Environnent Bio-Psycho-Social. Paris, Impression SPPI, 1996.

21 Haustgen T, Akiskal H: French antecedents of contemporary concepts in the American Psychiatric Association's classification of bipolar (mood) disorders. J Affect Disord 2006;96:149–163.

Joseph Westermeyer, MD, PhD
Department of Psychiatry, University of Minnesota
Mental Health Service, Minneapolis VA Medical Center
Minneapolis, MN 55417 (USA)
E-Mail weste010@umn.edu

Alarcón RD (ed): Cultural Psychiatry.
Adv Psychosom Med. Basel, Karger, 2013, vol 33, pp 64–74 (DOI: 10.1159/000350057)

Transcultural Aspects of Somatic Symptoms in the Context of Depressive Disorders

Issa P. Bagayogo[a] · Alejandro Interian[b, c] · Javier I. Escobar[a, b]

[a]Office of Global Health, UMDNJ – Robert Wood Johnson Medical School, New Brunswick, N.J.,
[b]Department of Psychiatry, UMDNJ – Robert Wood Johnson Medical School, Piscataway, N.J. and
[c]VA New Jersey Health Care System, Mental Health and Behavioral Sciences, Lyons, N.J., USA

Abstract

Somatic symptoms are a common presentation of mental disorders or psychological distress world-wide, and may often coexist with depressive and anxiety symptoms, thus accounting for what might be the most frequent psychiatric syndrome in primary care. Indeed, physical symptoms accompanying the clinical presentations of a variety of mental disorders may be considered as universal 'idioms of distress' that may vary across cultures, depending on attitudes and explanations embedded in each one of them. These variations in symptom presentations are the result of various interacting factors that ultimately determine how individuals identify and classify bodily sensations, perceive illness, and seek medical attention. This chapter examines the impact of culture on the experiencing of somatic symptoms, based on an inclusive review of the topic from ethnic, nosological, clinical and social perspectives. Particular attention is paid to the association of somatic symptoms with mood symptoms, since depressive disorders appear to be the most common, costly and disabling psychiatric entities worldwide. The review shows that racial/ethnic variations in somatic symptoms in the context of depression are common, and seem to be related to depression severity. Sociocultural factors, particularly stigma, may influence the unique emphasis placed on somatic symptoms within depression, and may account for some racial/ethnic differences in somatic symptom reporting.

Somatic symptoms are a truly kaleidoscopic component of many medical and psychiatric entities. While research efforts are duly oriented towards the determination of underlying physical (biochemical, pathophysiological or pharmacological) substrates, their meaning, impact and explanations as part of a human being's suffering belong to the sociocultural component of every pathological event, and are also the subject of numerous heuristic inquiries. This chapter examines precisely the impact of culture on the experiencing of somatic symptoms, and includes a comprehensive review of the topic from ethnic, nosological, clinical and social perspectives. The literature on the subject may not be voluminous, but shows clear leads towards valid theoretical interpretations and effective therapeutic interventions.

Thus, a major aim of this review is to strongly suggest that 'culture' – the set of values, attitudes, beliefs and expectations shared by a group of people – may ultimately influence the formation and presentations of symptoms in response to distress. Kleinman [1] was among the first to articulate the now well-accepted adage that in most cultures, the transformation of personal/social 'distress' into somatic complaints is actually the norm. Historian Edward Shorter took this view further, and posited that culture influences symptoms presentation in a manner that only the 'socially correct' forms of proper behavior are exhibited. Thus, individuals would tend to display those symptoms that are accepted and understood by society and its physicians.

A Brief History of Somatic Symptoms and Disorders in DSM

Somatic symptoms are a common representation of mental disorders or psychological distress worldwide. However, they rarely appear alone – indeed, a triad of depressive, anxiety and somatic symptoms may be the most frequent psychiatric syndrome in primary care [3–5]. In the Diagnostic and Statistical Manual (DSM) system of the American Psychiatric Association (APA), the classification of these somatic presentations has evolved over time, starting in the first two editions (DSM-I and DSM-II) with the historically relevant and traditional diagnoses of hysteria and hypochondriasis. While hypochondriasis was retained in the operational DSM-III and DSM-IV criteria for 'somatoform' disorders, hysteria became 'somatization disorder', a simple account of unexplained symptoms originating in many organ systems but already lacking in the florid, yet unsubstantiated psychodynamic meanings nourished by the Freudian doctrine. This counting went down from 14 or more symptoms in DSM-III to 5 or more in DSM-IV, including specific subtypes or variants such as pain and pseudoneurological manifestations. DSM-IV also created the broad category of 'undifferentiated' somatization disorder.

The delineation of 'somatoform' disorders required the presence of medically unexplained symptoms, a clinical judgment that proved to be quite difficult to articulate, an unreliable concept that reinforced the mind/body dualism, and was not well accepted by patients who felt the clinician's opinion was that the symptoms were not authentic, and/or insinuating that it was 'all in their head.' Using the DSM-III and DSM-IV criteria sets, somatization disorder appeared to be extremely rare in clinics and communities, was rarely used by psychiatrists and even less so by other medical specialists. DSM-5, the newest official diagnostic system represents a drastic change, reframing these disorders as 'somatic symptom disorders'. The changes in DSM-5 do not focus only on symptoms, but also on their impact on emotions, cognition, and behavior. The following sections present a review of literature contributions examining somatic presentations characterized by high levels of physical symptoms. Particular attention will be paid to their association with mood symptoms as well-known depressive disorders appear to be the most frequent, costly and disabling psychiatric entities worldwide.

Somatic Symptoms in Different Ethnic Groups

Culture-Specific Somatic Symptoms

Physical symptoms accompanying the clinical presentations of a variety of mental disorders may be considered a sort of universal 'idioms of distress' [1]. However, they may vary between different cultures, depending on attitudes and explanations [6–8] embedded in each one of them (including stigma). These cultural variations in symptom presentations are the result of various contextual, interacting factors that somehow determine how individuals identify and classify bodily sensations, perceive illness, and seek medical attention. In the case of common medical conditions, symptom presentations, medical explanations and interventions vary significantly even in Westernized societies. Payer [9, 10] described that in the United States and Canada, there is a focus on immunologically based symptoms such as 'viruses', 'environmental diseases' or 'multiple chemical sensitivities', while in Germany the emphasis is on 'poor circulation', 'low blood pressure' or *herzinsuffizienz* ('weak heart'). In England, there is excessive concern about 'bowel problems' such as constipation and red blotches on the skin ('chilblain'), whereas in France, 'liver crises' and a condition called 'adult spasmophilia' that include symptoms of hyperventilation, fatigue, dizziness, cramps and palpitations, are rather common.

In a review by the senior author (J.I.E.) [11], it was described that in Latin America and the Caribbean, a unique repertoire of somatoform and dissociative states (trance, possessions) has been reported for years. Examples include *ataque de nervios, susto, espanto, duende* and *mal de ojo.* Of note, somatizing/hypochondriac features co-presented with major depression amongst certain populations [11]. Interestingly, the most common somatic symptoms reported worldwide are gastrointestinal complaints and abnormal skin sensations, according to the ICD-10 manual.

Somatic Symptoms and Depressive Disorders

Some differences in the phenomenology of highly prevalent somatic symptoms accompanying depressive disorders across racial and ethnic groups have been reported. In turn, the assessment and treatment of depression with more or less abundant somatic symptoms remain unsatisfactory, particularly in primary care settings, probably the first stop in the help-seeking journey of these patients. In addition to complicating the presenting psychopathology, somatic symptoms negatively impact treatment response and prognosis. Much remains unknown regarding this clinical constellation because large-scale studies have often neglected somatic presentations.

Racial/Ethnic Influences of Somatic Symptoms on Depressive Disorders
The vast majority of studies conducted after the publication of DSM-IV indicate that somatic symptom reporting within depression was more commonly observed among racial/ethnic minorities in the US, compared to white non-Hispanic populations. Representative studies of patient samples carrying somatic manifestations within a depressive picture in different racial/ethnic groups are examined below.

Asians. Studies on depression among Chinese populations, without a cross-cultural comparative design, show quite prominent somatic symptoms. In one of them, 76% of Chinese American primary care patients with depression had chief complaints centered on somatic symptoms [12]. These findings were replicated in a study overseas, in Guangzhou, China, which showed that among patients who visited hospital clinics, somatic complaints were highly associated with depression and anxiety [13]. Similar results were found in a study in India, which found that somatic complaints were quite prevalent in subjects presenting with first-episode depression [14]. In studies among Asian samples employing a cross-cultural comparative design, evidence shows either greater numbers or salience of somatic symptoms in the clinical presentations, or greater attribution of somatic causes of depression. One study compared outpatient psychiatric samples with depression in Toronto (Caucasians) and China [15]; the results revealed that the Chinese patients experienced more somatic and less psychological symptoms on both, spontaneous problem report and structured clinical interviews. A comparison of college students from Japan and the US showed that the former reported greater levels of somatic distress [16]. The authors also reported a greater association between depression severity score and somatic symptoms endorsement among Japanese students (0.57 vs. 0.19, respectively).

A study comparing Malaysian Chinese and Australian Caucasian outpatients with depression found that the former were more likely to spontaneously describe somatic symptoms [17]. Specifically, 60% of Malaysian Chinese nominated a somatic symptom, while the rate was only 13% among Australian Caucasians. Differences were also noted on a depression self-report inventory. A primary care-based study in Australia compared Chinese patients who spoke mostly Cantonese or Mandarin, Chinese who spoke English, and Australian Caucasian patients [18]. Participants were presented with a list of depressive symptoms and asked to attribute or identify the cause of the symptoms (psychological, somatic, normal, other). The Chinese-speaking Chinese patients were more likely than those of the other two groups to offer a somatizing attribution for fatigue, as well as less likely to offer a psychological attribution. These differences did not emerge between English-speaking Chinese and the Australian Caucasians. This study suggested that level of acculturation among the Chinese subjects accounted for the findings, as English-speaking Chinese were quite similar to non-Chinese patients.

In a different geographic and ethnic scenario, a study in Hawaii compared the depression scores of Caucasian, Native Hawaiians and Japanese American community respondents using the CES-D [19]. Native Hawaiians scored higher than Caucasians on the somatic symptom subscale. There were no differences between Japanese American and Caucasians.

US Latinos. Studies on US Latino populations also document a tendency for greater somatic symptoms reported as part of depressive occurrences. In the STAR*D Study, a large-scale trial examining the effectiveness of sequenced antidepressant treatment, Latinos were 40% more likely to report pain symptoms together with their depression [20]. A study by the senior author using a primary care sample found that Central American immigrants had higher rates of abridged somatization (30%), relative to non-Latino Whites and Mexican Immigrants (17–22%), though the statistical significance of this difference disappeared after adjusting for demographic variables [21]. Another study found that Puerto Rican outpatients with depression reported more somatic symptoms on the Brief Symptom Inventory, compared with non-Latino Whites [22]. Similarly, a study focusing on female outpatients with depression reported that Latinas endorsed more somatic symptoms than non-Latino White women [23].

African-Americans. In our review of research conducted in the US, we found only a handful of studies showing that somatic symptom reporting was more common among Africa-American populations. Using data from a randomized controlled trial for major depression, Brown et al. [24] found that 38% of African-Americans met the criteria for abridged somatization, compared with 25% of non-Latino Whites. These authors conducted another evaluation of randomized trial data and found that African-Americans were rated as carrying more severe somatic items recorded by the HAM-D, relative to non-Latino Whites [25]. African-American women receiving outpatient treatment for depression reported more somatic complaints than non-Latino White women [23]. Also, the STAR*D study found that African-Americans with depression were 34% more likely to report pain symptoms [20].

There are limited data on somatic symptom presentations among black patients from other nations. The World Health Organization (WHO) International Collaborative Study of Psychological Problems in General Health Care provides some data on primary care patients from Nigeria. Analysis of these data showed that, out of 15 sites, Nigeria ranked third in most frequent and spontaneous reporting of somatic symptoms, while also meeting criteria for major depression [26]. The Nigerian site ranked ninth in terms of reporting the most medically unexplained symptoms, and fourth in terms of denying two key psychological symptoms (depressed mood and feelings of guilt/worthlessness) although still meeting criteria for major depression. However, it should be noted that while the WHO studies did seem to show considerable racial/ethnic variation in somatic symptom reporting, a clear pattern to the variation did not emerge vis-à-vis non-Western, non-Caucasian patients).

Other Studies. It should be mentioned that a different pattern, i.e. an actual lack of racial/ethnic influences on somatic symptom- reporting are suggested by a few studies. For example, among Asian subjects, one study comparing community samples from South Korea and the US found no differences in somatization, which was defined as the reporting of physical symptoms in the absence of a general medical condition [27]. Another study compared college students in China, Chinese American US students, and Caucasian US college students on the somatization factor scale of the CES-D [28]. The results showed that the Chinese students had lower somatization factor scores in comparison to the Chinese Americans and the US Caucasians. Also, an analysis of data from the Epidemiological Catchment Area (ECA) study showed that rates of somatization disorder were lower among Asians relative to Caucasians [29]. However, this study did not examine somatic symptoms within depressive diagnoses. Lack of racial/ethnic variability of somatic symptoms was also reported among African-Americans in one study [30]. The authors showed that there was no difference on the somatic factor scale of the HAM-D between African-Americans and non-Latino white patients with depression.

Overall, this literature review shows that somatic symptoms are commonly represented within depression across racial and ethnic groups. Also, the majority of studies do indicate racial/ethnic variation, as Latino and non-Caucasian populations seem to report somatic symptoms slightly more so than Caucasian ones. This pattern is most consistently seen in studies using clinical samples. The racial/ethnic variation in somatic symptom reporting is a general pattern and certainly not one that occurs without exception.

Understanding Racial/Ethnic Variations in Somatic Symptom Reporting within Depression

Relationship between Severity of Depression, Level of Distress and Somatic Presentations
On the basis of studies reporting sufficiently comprehensive data, we examined whether or not the report of higher rates of somatic symptoms was significantly associated with greater overall distress in different racial/ethnic groups.

For example, among African-American patients with depression and higher rates of abridged somatization, generally more severe levels of depression and psychosocial stressors were also apparent [24].

In Asian patients, a study showing that Native Hawaiian community respondents who scored higher than US Caucasians and Japanese Americans on the somatic factor of the CES-D, also showed higher levels of overall severity of depression [19]; since no differences in somatic symptoms were present between Japanese Americans and US Caucasians, these groups did not differ on overall depression severity. Also, Japanese college students reporting more somatic symptoms than US Caucasians, were found to experience more severe overall levels of depression [16]. Studies using clinical samples in South Korea found that the presence of painful physical symptoms was associated with greater depression severity and lower quality of life [31, 32]. Similar results were found in an observational study on depressed patients from China, Hong Kong, Korea, Malaysia, Singapore and Taiwan [33].

Among US Latinos, Myers et al. [23] found greater somatic symptom reporting among African-Americans and Latino women; these two groups were also more severely depressed than Caucasian females. Marginal evidence for greater severity was demonstrated in a study showing that Puerto Rican patients with depression reported more somatic symptoms than Caucasians [22]. Specifically, these results showed a trend for Puerto Ricans to report more overall symptoms, but no differences on another global severity index. In an analysis of the STAR*D data set, increasing severity of pain symptoms was associated with greater disease burden and higher depression among African-American and Hispanic patients [34].

However, it is also important to acknowledge some studies that do not demonstrate these patterns. The STAR*D Study reported greater pain complaints among Latinos and African Americans, even after adjusting for depression severity [20, 34]. Other analyses on this dataset showed that Latinos and African-American were not clearly more severely ill than non-Latino Whites [35]. As well, a study reporting greater somatic symptom reporting in US vs. China college students, failed to find corresponding severity differences [28]. Similarly, analysis of a randomized controlled trial dataset found no differences in somatic symptoms between black women (US-born, African-born, Caribbean-born) despite considerable differences in rates of depression [36]. Finally, an analysis of epidemiological data showed that Latinos with depression reported more pain than non-Latino Whites with depression [37]. This pattern, however, occurred despite equal rates of depression.

In summary, a general perspective on these results provides evidence of some racial/ethnic variations on somatic symptom reporting, which corresponds with differences in severity [16, 19, 22–24, 31–33]. However, a major weakness of these studies is that many were not primarily designed to answer this question directly and, therefore, provide a tenuous glimpse of whether racial/ethnic variations decisively account for severity. Furthermore, there are other results that fail to correspond to this pattern [20, 28, 35–37], suggesting that perhaps additional factors need to be accounted for.

'Stigma' and Somatic Presentations

There are a handful of studies that document the relationship between stigma related to mental health problems and somatic symptom reporting, as well as racial/ethnic variations in depression stigma. A study using data from the Chinese American Psychiatric Epidemiological Survey examined how Chinese American community respondents rated the social disruptiveness of depression, anxiety, and somatoform disorders [38]. The results showed that depression (84.5%) and anxiety (81.1%) were most rated as socially disruptive, while somatoform disorders were rated the least (55.2%). Another study examined psychiatric outpatients in India, diagnosed with a depressive disorder, a somatoform disorder or both [39]. Patients diagnosed only with somatoform disorders reported significantly lower stigma scores than those with depression only. Stigma scores were also positively correlated to HAMD scores. In India, another study focusing on psychiatric outpatients showed participants with greater stigma concerns reporting more somatic symptoms vis-à-vis psychological ones [40]. Using a convenience sample of European and Chinese Americans rating clinical vignettes of depression, Georg Hsu et al. [41] reported higher stigma ratings among the latter. Furthermore, in a comparison of psychiatric outpatients with depression in China versus Toronto, Canada, Chinese patients reported greater levels of mental health stigma [15], associated with increased reporting of both psychological and somatic symptoms.

In the US, racial/ethnic minority women were far more likely to endorse stigma concerns, relative to Caucasian women [42]. Immigrant Latinas were 26% more likely, immigrant African women were 39% more likely and Caribbean born women were 45% more likely to endorse them compared to Caucasians. While this specific study demonstrated the cross-racial/ethnic variability of mental health stigma, it did not report how this data was related to depressive versus somatic symptoms. Collectively, the data provides some evidence for the differential social impact of somatic versus psychological symptoms; such a differential impact can reinforce symptom experiences in a way that shapes their final clinical presentation.

Illness Models
Somatic symptom presentation may also be influenced by patients' illness models. As specified by Kirmayer and Sartorius [43], a range of factors can serve to amplify the somatic sensations that accompany the individual's experience. Amplification may occur via complex feedback loops that are associated with increased anxiety/concern over somatic symptoms, illness-related behaviors related to the somatic symptom, and activation of physiological pathways that further exacerbate the symptoms [44–46]. Many of the potential feedback factors are tied to social influences. For example, the reactions of others within a patient's social network can reinforce different aspects of the illness experience, which relates to the stigma influences or factors described above. Patients' models of illness also relate to a number of feedback loops, as the individual's interpretations of symptoms essentially influence his/her attention to the symptoms. For instance, increased attention to a symptom is more likely to follow if such symptom is perceived to be related to a serious condition. Such interpretations also influence the emotional reaction to that symptom.

Thus, the predominance of somatic illness models is likely to shape the symptom presentation of depressive disorders via emphasis on somatic symptoms. These illness models would include culturally based models such as the Dhat syndrome and *ataque de nervios* [47–49]. One study, for example, showed that *ataque de nervios* was related to the presentation of unexplained neurological symptoms [49]. In addition, a series of studies have demonstrated that the cultural notions of illness are associated with symptom amplification that, in turn, leads to panic attacks or similar pictures [50–55]. One study focused on Vietnamese patients who experienced orthostatically induced panic attacks, found that culturally based catastrophic cognitions and trauma associations were related to the severity of these attacks [54]. Together, these studies provide a small level of evidence illustrating the association between culturally influenced notions of illness and symptom presentation. To reiterate it, cultural notions of illness in depression may influence feedback loops in ways that amplify somatic symptoms. However, firm conclusions on these topics could only be arrived at through needed additional research.

Conclusions

As a whole, this review shows a tendency for Latino, Black and Asian populations with depression to emphasize somatic symptoms in their clinical presentations. This pattern is more likely observed among clinical population when compared with community-based samples. However, it would be erroneous to consider somatic symptom reporting within depression to be a unique Latino or non-Caucasian occurrence since high levels have also been reported among Caucasians populations [20].

Racial/ethnic variations in somatic symptoms may at times relate to greater severity of depression. However, this is not always the case, as other factors need to be considered to fully understand the different levels of these 'somatization' phenomena in clinical depression.

Sociocultural factors, particularly stigma related to depressive disorder, may influence the unique emphasis placed on somatic symptoms within depression, and may account for some racial/ethnic differences in somatic symptom reporting. The impact of existing illness models in this context represents an emerging field of study in need of more focused and intensive studies. In particular, research works should directly assess this issue via culturally comparative designs that examine illness model distinctions and their relationship to well characterized and measured somatic symptom presentations.

References

1 Kleinman A: Anthropology and psychiatry. The role of culture in cross-cultural research on illness. Br J Psychiatry 1987;151:447–454.
2 Shorter E: A History of Psychiatry. New York, Free Press, 1997.
3 Lowe B, Spitzer RL, Williams JB, Mussell M, Schellberg D, Kroenke K: Depression, anxiety and somatization in primary care: syndrome overlap and functional impairment. Gen Hosp Psychiatry 2008;30:191–199.
4 Gureje O, Simon GE, Ustun TB, Goldberg DP: Somatization in cross-cultural perspective: a World Health Organization study in primary care. Am J Psychiatry 1997;154:989–995.
5 Toft T, Fink P, Oernboel E, Christensen K, Frostholm L, Olesen F: Mental disorders in primary care: prevalence and co-morbidity among disorders. Results from the functional illness in primary care (FIP) study. Psychol Med 2005;35:1175–1184.

6 Fabrega H Jr: Psychiatric diagnosis. A cultural perspective. J Nerv Ment Dis 1987;175:383–394.

7 Kirmayer LJ: Culture affect and somatization. Transcult Res Rev 1984;21:159–188.

8 Kleinman A: Culture, depression and the new cross-cultural psychiatry. Soc Sci Med 1977;11:3–11.

9 Payer L: Medicine and Culture. New York, Henry Holt, 1989.

10 Payer L: Borderline cases: How medical practice reflects national culture. Sciences 1990:38–42.

11 Escobar JI: Transcultural aspects of dissociative and somatoform disorders. Psychiatr Clins North Am 1995;18:555–569.

12 Yeung A, Chang D, Gresham RL Jr, Nierenberg AA, Fava M: Illness beliefs of depressed Chinese American patients in primary care. J Nerv Ment Dis 2004; 192:324–327.

13 Zhu C, Ou L, Geng Q, Zhang M, Ye R, Chen J, et al: Association of somatic symptoms with depression and anxiety in clinical patients of general hospitals in Guangzhou, China. Gen Hosp Psychiatry 2012;34: 113–120.

14 Grover S, Kumar V, Chakrabarti S, Hollikatti P, Singh P, Tyagi S, et al: Prevalence and type of functional somatic complaints in patients with first-episode depression. East Asian Arch Psychiatry 2012; 22:146–153.

15 Ryder AG, Yang J, Zhu X, Yao S, Yi J, Heine SJ, et al: The cultural shaping of depression: somatic symptoms in China, psychological symptoms in North America? J Abnorm Psychol 2008;117:300–313.

16 Arnault DS, Sakamoto S, Moriwaki A: Somatic and depressive symptoms in female Japanese and American students: a preliminary investigation. Transcult Psychiatry 2006;43:275–286.

17 Parker G, Cheah YC, Roy K: Do the Chinese somatize depression? A cross-cultural study. Soc Psychiatry Psychiatr Epidemiol 2001;36:287–293.

18 Parker G, Chan B, Tully L, Eisenbruch M: Depression in the Chinese: the impact of acculturation. Psychol Med 2005;35:1475–1483.

19 Kanazawa A, White PM, Hampson SE: Ethnic variation in depressive symptoms in a community sample in Hawaii. Cult Divers Ethnic Minority Psychol 2007;13:35–44.

20 Husain MM, Rush AJ, Trivedi MH, McClintock SM, Wisniewski SR, Davis L, et al: Pain in depression: STAR*D study findings. J Psychosom Res 2007;63: 113–122.

21 Escobar JI, Waitzkin H, Silver RC, Gara M, Holman A: Abridged somatization: a study in primary care. Psychosom Med 1998;60:466–472.

22 Coelho VL, Strauss ME, Jenkins JH: Expression of symptomatic distress by Puerto Rican and Euro-American patients with depression and schizophrenia. J Nerv Ment Dis 1998;186:477–483.

23 Myers HF, Lesser I, Rodriguez N, Mira CB, Hwang WC, Camp C, et al: Ethnic differences in clinical presentation of depression in adult women. Cult Divers Ethnic Minority Psychol 2002;8:138–156.

24 Brown C, Schulberg HC, Madonia MJ: Clinical presentations of major depression by African Americans and whites in primary medical care practice. J Affect Disord 1996;41:181–191.

25 Brown C, Schulberg HC, Sacco D, Perel JM, Houck PR: Effectiveness of treatments for major depression in primary medical care practice: a post hoc analysis of outcomes for African American and white patients. J Affect Disord 1999;53:185–192.

26 Simon GE, VonKorff M, Piccinelli M, Fullerton C, Ormel J: An international study of the relation between somatic symptoms and depression. N Engl J Med 1999;341:1329–1335.

27 Keyes CL, Ryff CD: Somatization and mental health: a comparative study of the idiom of distress hypothesis. Soc Sci Med 2003;57:1833–1845.

28 Yen S, Robins CJ, Lin N: A cross-cultural comparison of depressive symptom manifestation: China and the United States. J Consult Clin Psychol 2000; 68:993–999.

29 Zhang AY, Snowden LR: Ethnic characteristics of mental disorders in five US communities. Cult Divers Ethnic Minority Psychol 1999;5:134–146.

30 Wohi M, Lesser I, Smith M: Clinical presentations of depression in African American and white outpatients. Cult Divers Ment Health 1997;3:279–284.

31 Bahk WM, Park S, Jon DI, Yoon BH, Min KJ, Hong JP: Relationship between painful physical symptoms and severity of depressive symptomatology and suicidality. Psychiatry Res 2011;189:357–361.

32 Lee MS, Yum SY, Hong JP, Yoon SC, Noh JS, Lee KH, et al: Association between painful physical symptoms and clinical outcomes in Korean patients with major depressive disorder: a three-month observational study. Psychiatry Invest 2009;6:255–263.

33 Ang QQ, Wing YK, He Y, Sulaiman AH, Chiu NY, Shen YC, et al: Association between painful physical symptoms and clinical outcomes in East Asian patients with major depressive disorder: a 3-month prospective observational study. Int J Clin Pract 2009;63:1041–1049.

34 Leuchter AF, Husain MM, Cook IA, Trivedi MH, Wisniewski SR, Gilmer WS, et al: Painful physical symptoms and treatment outcome in major depressive disorder: a STAR*D (Sequenced Treatment Alternatives to Relieve Depression) report. Psychol Med 2010;40:239–251.

35 Lesser IM, Castro DB, Gaynes BN, Gonzalez J, Rush AJ, Alpert JE, et al: Ethnicity/race and outcome in the treatment of depression: results from STAR*D. Med Care 2007;45:1043–1051.

36 Miranda J, Siddique J, Belin TR, Kohn-Wood LP: Depression prevalence in disadvantaged young black women: African and Caribbean immigrants compared to US-born African Americans. Soc Psychiatry Psychiatr Epidemiol 2005;40:253–258.

37 Hernandez A, Sachs-Ericsson N: Ethnic differences in pain reports and the moderating role of depression in a community sample of Hispanic and Caucasian participants with serious health problems. Psychosom Med 2006;68:121–128.

38 Kung WW, Lu PC: How symptom manifestations affect help seeking for mental health problems among Chinese Americans. J Nerv Ment Dis 2008;196:46–54.

39 Raguram R, Weiss MG, Channabasavanna SM, Devins GM: Stigma, depression, and somatization in South India. Am J Psychiatry 1996;153:1043–1049.

40 Rao D, Young M, Raguram R: Culture, somatization, and psychological distress: symptom presentation in South Indian patients from a public psychiatric hospital. Psychopathology 2007;40:349–355.

41 Georg Hsu LK, Wan YM, Chang H, Summergrad P, Tsang BY, Chen H: Stigma of depression is more severe in Chinese Americans than Caucasian Americans. Psychiatry 2008;71:210–218.

42 Nadeem E, Lange JM, Edge D, Fongwa M, Belin T, Miranda J: Does stigma keep poor young immigrant and U.S.-born Black and Latina women from seeking mental health care? Psychiatr Serv 2007;58:1547–1554.

43 Kirmayer LJ, Sartorius N: Cultural models and somatic syndromes. Psychosom Med 2007;69:832–840.

44 Dimsdale JE, Dantzer R: A biological substrate for somatoform disorders: importance of pathophysiology. Psychosom Med 2007;69:850–854.

45 Kirmayer LJ, Groleau D, Looper KJ, Dao MD: Explaining medically unexplained symptoms. Can J Psychiatry 2004;49:663–672.

46 Woolfolk RL, Allen LA: Treating Somatization. A Cognitive-Behavioral Approach. New York, Guilford Press, 2007.

47 Guarnaccia PJ, Rubio-Stipec M, Canino G: Ataques de nervios in the Puerto Rican Diagnostic Interview Schedule: the impact of cultural categories on psychiatric epidemiology. Cult Med Psychiatry 1989;13:275–295.

48 Ranjith G, Mohan R: Dhat syndrome as a functional somatic syndrome: developing a sociosomatic model. Psychiatry 2006;69:142–150.

49 Interian A, Guarnaccia PJ, Vega WA, Gara MA, Like RC, Escobar JI, et al: The relationship between ataque de nervios and unexplained neurological symptoms: a preliminary analysis. J Nerv Ment Dis 2005;193:32–39.

50 Hinton D, Hinton S, Pham T, Chau H, Tran M: 'Hit by the wind' and temperature-shift panic among Vietnamese refugees. Transcult Psychiatry 2003;40:342–376.

51 Hinton D, Pich V, Chhean D, Pollack M: Olfactory-triggered panic attacks among Khmer refugees: a contextual approach. Transcult Psychiatry 2004;41:155–199.

52 Hinton DE, Chhean D, Fama JM, Pollack MH, McNally RJ: Gastrointestinal-focused panic attacks among Cambodian refugees: associated psychopathology, flashbacks, and catastrophic cognitions. J Anxiety Disord 2007;21:42–58.

53 Hinton DE, Chhean D, Pich V, Um K, Fama JM, Pollack MH: Neck-focused panic attacks among Cambodian refugees; a logistic and linear regression analysis. J Anxiety Disord 2006;20:119–138.

54 Hinton DE, Hinton L, Tran M, Nguyen L, Hsia C, Pollack MH: Orthostatically induced panic attacks among Vietnamese refugees: associated psychopathology, flashbacks, and catastrophic cognitions. Depression Anxiety 2006;23:113–115.

55 Hinton DE, Pich V, Chhean D, Pollack MH, Barlow DH: Olfactory-triggered panic attacks among Cambodian refugees attending a psychiatric clinic. Gen Hosp Psychiatry 2004;26:390–397.

Javier I. Escobar, MD, MSc
University of Medicine and Dentistry of New Jersey-Robert Wood Johnson Medical School
Clinical Academic Building, Room 7038, 125 Paterson Street
New Brunswick, NJ 08901 (USA)
E-Mail escobaja@umdnj.edu

Alarcón RD (ed): Cultural Psychiatry.
Adv Psychosom Med. Basel, Karger, 2013, vol 33, pp 75–87 (DOI: 10.1159/000348735)

Culture and Demoralization in Psychotherapy

John M. de Figueiredo[a] · Sara Gostoli[b]

[a]Department of Psychiatry, Yale University School of Medicine, New Haven, Conn., USA;
[b]Department of Psychology, University of Bologna, Bologna, Italy

Abstract

In most societies, members of a culture have attempted to help each other in times of trouble with various types of healing methods. Demoralization – an individual experience related to a group phenomenon – responds to certain elements shared by all psychotherapies. This article has three objectives: (1) to review the theoretical background leading to our current views on culture and demoralization in psychotherapy, (2) to discuss the methodological challenges faced in the cross-cultural study of demoralization and psychotherapy, and (3) to describe the clinical applications and research prospects of this area of inquiry. Demoralization follows a shattering of the individual's assumptive world and it is different from homeostatic responses to a stressful situation or from depressive disorders. Only a few comparative studies of this construct across cultures have been undertaken. The presentation of distress may vary widely from culture to culture and even within the same culture. To avoid 'category fallacy', it is important to understand the idioms of distress peculiar to a cultural group. A cultural psychiatrist or psychotherapist would have to identify patient's values and sentiments, reconstruct his/her personal and collective ambient worlds, and only then study demoralization. The limitations of our current diagnostic systems have resulted in methodological challenges. Cultural clinicians should consider using a combination of both 'clinimetric' and 'perspectivistic' approaches in order to arrive at a diagnosis and identify the appropriate intervention. The presenting problem has to be understood in the context of the patient's individual, social and cultural background, and patients unfamiliar with Western-type psychotherapies have to be prepared to guide their own expectations before the former are used. Future research should identify the gaps in knowledge on the effectiveness of cultural psychotherapy at reversing or preventing demoralization.

Copyright © 2013 S. Karger AG, Basel

Theoretical Background

From time immemorial, in many, if not all, societies members of a culture have attempted to help each other in times of trouble. In the so-called 'primitive' or 'pre-industrialized' societies, such attempts have taken the form of indigenous healing practices. These include approaches such as trance-based practices, religious healing ceremonies, divination, fortune-telling and meditation exercises. Though commonly identified as 'primitive', such practices are also found in developed societies, but unlike some other healing methods, they are 'culture-embedded' [1]. Other practices are influenced by beliefs commonly held in certain cultures at a given time; they are often applicable to a limited group of patients or a specific disorder. Examples are Mesmerism, Naikkan therapy, and Morita therapy, and they are appropriately called 'culture-influenced unique' healing methods. A third group are the mainstream psychotherapies, such as psychoanalysis and other psychodynamic therapies, client-centered psychotherapy, behavior therapy, cognitive and cognitive-behavioral therapies, and marital, family and group therapies. These mainstream therapies are also influenced by culture and their acceptability may vary depending on the historical and cultural contexts. This classification of psychotherapies, first proposed by Tseng, enables us to understand how, in the Western world, the practice of psychotherapy, like the practice of medicine, moved from a religious and philosophical foundation to a secular and scientific orientation [2, 3].

Until recently, the common ground of all healing methods and the effective ingredients of their success had remained poorly understood. Our current understanding of the theory of psychotherapy as it relates to culture came largely from the seminal work of Jerome D. Frank, Alexander H. Leighton and Karl Jaspers. In addition, the distinction between signs and symbols, first proposed by Ernest Cassirer, and the concept of *Umwelt* (a German word that may be roughly translated as 'ambient world') introduced by Jakob von Uexkull, an ethologist, are relevant to the conceptualization of cultural aspects of psychotherapy [4–10].

In his book, *Persuasion and Healing*, first published in 1961, Jerome D. Frank noted that persons who seek psychotherapy, irrespective of their diagnostic label, are 'deprived of spirit or courage, disheartened, bewildered, and thrown into disorder or confusion'. He referred to their state of mind as 'demoralization', and proposed that demoralization responds to the elements shared by all psychotherapies. He further suggested that demoralization involves a breakdown of the demoralized person's assumptive world [4].

Several different definitions and criteria for demoralization have been proposed (for a review, see de Figueiredo [11]). Actually, demoralization had been previously observed in different clinical settings and received different names. For example, a type of existential despair or loss of 'fighting spirit' had been noticed by Engel in patients with medical illness and called 'giving up-given up complex' [12, 13]; acute demoralization was recognized by Caplan [14] in the emergency departments and called 'crisis', and chronic demoralization had been seen in patients with schizophrenia by Gruenberg [15] who called it 'social breakdown syndrome'.

How does demoralization, an individual experience, relate to a group phenomenon and a process such as culture? The answer to this crucial question became clear when Leighton [5] introduced the concept of 'sentiments' and defined them as relatively stable components of personality made up of attitudes and values. Attitudes, in turn, are relatively stable combinations of beliefs, emotions and wants (i.e. the 'desired' potential behaviors). While wants are 'desired', values are 'desirable'. According to Kluckhohn and Strodtbeck [16], a value is 'a conception (explicit or implicit, distinctive of an individual or characteristic of a group) of the desirable which influences the selection from available modes, means and ends of action'.

According to Kluckhohn and Strodtbeck [16] values are oriented towards five common human problems for which human beings at all times must find solutions. The type of solution adopted defines the person's value orientation. The five value orientations are time (past, present, future), human activity (being, being-in-becoming, doing), relationship to other people (lineal, collateral, individualistic), relationship to nature (subjugation to nature, harmony with nature, mastery over nature), and belief about innate human nature (evil, neutral or mixture of good and evil, good) [17]. Since values are part of sentiments, the same five orientations could be applied to sentiments.

A third concept that enabled us to understand the relationship of psychotherapy and culture is that of 'meaningful connections', first introduced by Jaspers [6]. 'Meaningful connections' are idiosyncratic interpretations of links among events in a person's life story. As Frank and Frank [4, p. 24] elegantly stated, 'just as nature is said to abhor a physical vacuum, so the human mind abhors a vacuum of meaning'. Cassirer [7–9] distinguished two types of vehicles of meaning: signs and symbols. While signs denote and present, symbols connote and represent. In operant conditioning, the sound of a bell is a sign that announces to the animal that food is coming. A red traffic light is a sign for the traffic to stop, but the color red may be a symbol of war for a combat veteran. In this instance, the traffic sign elicits a behavior, while the color red generates ideas and emotions. Signs are elicited by environmental cues; symbols are representations of ideas and emotions. As Cassirer noted, animals other than man cannot symbolize. It is the ability to symbolize that allows man to transmit ideas from one generation to the next creating a repository of knowledge called culture. This distinction between signs and symbols is critical for cross-cultural psychotherapy because words, as Cassirer noted, can be both signs and symbols. Signs and symbols can be studied objectively in terms of form, meaning, use, and function [18, p. 402].

The sentiments in a society are hierarchically organized, with some being more dominant than others. By means of symbols, members of a society share sentiments, some of which are dominant. A sentiment is called 'dominant' when the beliefs included in that sentiment (assumptions, expectations and values) refer to issues viewed as vital to the common good and survival of the members of a society. Dominant sentiments are called 'essential striving sentiments' by Leighton [5] whereas the symbols that represent dominant sentiments may be called 'dominant symbols'.

As stated above, according to Frank and Frank [4, p. 24], demoralization involves a breakdown of the assumptive world. Assumptions are subjective certainties (axioms or postulates); expectations are subjective likelihoods (probabilities). An assumptive world is a 'set of highly structured, complex, interacting values, expectations, and images of self and others that are closely related to emotional states and feelings'. In turn, a reformulation of 'assumptive world' led to the concept of *Umwelt* ('ambient world') to describe the perceptual world of a nonhuman animal [10]. While sentiments are subjective, they cannot be measured directly and can only be inferred, the symbols representing sentiments are objective and may be viewed as linked to each other by meaningful interconnections forming the *Umwelt*. A personal *Umwelt* may be defined as symbols representing a person's own sentiments, hierarchically organized by their degree of dominance, and the meaningful interconnections among those symbols at a given time [19]. It consists of meaningfully interconnected Lewinian fields [20]. A collective *Umwelt* is the common ground of all personal *Umwelten*, and consists of dominant sentiments and their meaningful interconnections [19].

The next important question is how to distinguish demoralization from 'normal', homeostatic responses to a stressful situation and from depressive disorders and other forms of diagnosable psychopathology. To draw the boundaries of demoralization, it has been proposed that it is a second-order construct and consists of nonspecific or specific distress and subjective incompetence [19, 21]. By generalizing and slightly modifying a definition proposed for cancer patients, distress may be defined as follows: 'An unpleasant emotional experience of a psychological, social, and/or spiritual nature that may interfere with the ability to cope effectively with a stressful situation. Distress extends along a spectrum, ranging from common nonpathological feelings of vulnerability, sadness, and fears to problems that can become disabling, such as depression, anxiety, panic, social isolation, and spiritual crisis' [22, 23]. Subjective incompetence is a self-perceived incapacity to perform tasks and express feelings deemed appropriate in a stressful situation, resulting in pervasive uncertainty and doubts about the future. When they occur by themselves, distress and subjective incompetence may be 'normal', i.e. non-pathological. Normal grief is an example of distress without subjective incompetence. Examples of subjective incompetence occurring without distress are the sense of uncertainty experienced by an immigrant newly arrived to his 'land of promise', or the sense of failing to meet our own expectations or those of others in a situation irrelevant to our self-esteem. When distress and subjective incompetence co-occur, their overlap initiates a cascade of events called demoralization [19, 21].

As the stressful situation persists or increases in severity, subjective incompetence becomes helplessness; some people who are helpless become hopeless; and some who are hopeless become suicidal. As Abramson et al. [24] noted, hopelessness always involves helplessness, i.e. hopelessness is a subset of helplessness, and, therefore, when hopelessness occurs, helplessness also occurs. Social support and perceived stress are the mediators of the co-occurrence of distress and subjective incompetence. When social support is strong (i.e. perceived as available and adequate) and perceived stress is low, distress and subjective incompetence do not occur together, the converse being true if social supports are weak and perceived stress is high.

Methodological Challenges

An important advance in the understanding of demoralization came from the studies of Dohrenwend et al. [25]. They noted that the content of psychiatric screening scales, including a scale that they had developed, was very similar to Frank's descriptions of the complaints of patients seeking outpatient psychotherapy. They confirmed what others before them had noted, namely that psychiatric screening scales measure a common underlying dimension to which they referred as 'demoralization'. Diagnostic criteria to assess demoralization in psychosomatic disorders and a corresponding scale, three other scales specifically designed to measure demoralization, and a scale to assess subjective incompetence are now available [26–31]. With these methods in place, a number of studies conducted in the United States, Canada, Europe, Israel, Australia and New Zealand have documented demoralization in both clinical populations and community samples. Of particular interest has been the demonstration that demoralization can be distinguished from depression among refugees and immigrants (for a review of these studies, see de Figueiredo [11]). The general conclusion from these studies is that demoralization can be a risk factor for the manifestation of psychopathology and certain physical illnesses, the prodromal phase of a mental disorder, or a trigger for exacerbation or recurrence of psychiatric distress symptoms.

Given the centrality of demoralization in psychiatry, it is surprising to note that comparative studies of this construct across nations and cultures have not yet been undertaken to any significant degree. Demoralization was documented in aboriginal communities, e.g. in Australia and in Canada, among refugees in New Zealand with depressive disorders who did not respond well to treatment, and among Bosnian refugees in Germany [32–37]. Instead, the focus of cross-national and cross-cultural research has been on depression. Such studies typically use predefined criteria to arrive at a diagnosis of a depressive disorder, and fail to recognize that a common human reaction to loss, frustration or disappointment is a combination of depression, anxiety, anger and other nonspecific symptoms of distress. Furthermore, although depressive disorders (e.g. depressive episode of bipolar disorder, major depressive disorder, or dysthymic disorder) and demoralization may co-exist, a fundamental difference separates them: if the motivation to get out of a predicament is viewed as a vector with a magnitude and a direction, demoralized individuals have the magnitude of motivation but lack the direction of action, the converse being true of individuals with depressive disorders. Also, the distinction between depression as a symptom and depression as a disorder is critical because demoralized individuals may experience symptoms of depression and other symptoms of distress, such as anxiety and anger, but they do not necessarily suffer from a diagnosable depressive disorder [38].

Case identification is essential in psychiatric epidemiology and clinical practice. In the absence of biological markers, case identification in psychiatry is achieved by the formulation of reliable diagnostic criteria. While there is no question that certain mental disorders (e.g. delirium, dementia, schizophrenia and bipolar disorder) are present worldwide, available evidence indicates that the presentation of distress and subjective incompetence may vary immensely from culture to culture and even within the same culture. It is, therefore, of the utmost importance to gain a clearer and deeper understanding of the idioms of distress and subjective incompetence peculiar to a cultural group before case identification is attempted [39]. The arbitrary use, in non-Western settings, of diagnostic categories developed in the West may lead to what Kleinman [40] called 'category fallacy', defined as 'the reification of one culture's diagnostic categories and their projection onto patients in another culture, where those categories lack coherence and their validity has not been established'. The establishment of standardized criteria for depressive disorders, even if valid and reliable, may result in the exclusion of alternative ways to react to loss, frustration and disappointment, a problem known as 'netting effect' [2, p. 321]. These alternative expressions and reactions would be captured if demoralization were assessed at the beginning of the diagnostic process. To complicate this even more, epidemiological studies have documented the extensive comorbidity of mental disorders, a result of such disorders being conceptualized as discrete entities [41]. Other factors such as progression of the disorder, overall severity, social support, perceived stress, resilience, and previous response to treatment also play a role in clinical decision making, but they are not adequately captured by our diagnostic systems [42, 43].

Clinical Applications

Psychotherapeutic Approaches
Psychotherapy was defined by Frank as the relief of demoralization in one or more persons by a trained professional using an approach based on a particular theory or paradigm [4]. Tseng [44] offered a broader definition he claimed was more suitable for cultural psychiatry: 'Psychotherapy is a special practice involving a designated healer (or therapist) and an identified client (or patient), with the particular purpose of solving a problem from which the client is suffering or promoting the health of the client's mind.' From his comparative study of the various modalities of psychotherapy, Frank [4, pp. 40–44] concluded that 'they all share at least four effective features: an emotionally charged, confiding relationship with a helping person (often with the participation of a group); a healing setting; a rationale, conceptual scheme, or myth that provides a plausible explanation for the patient's symptoms and prescribes a ritual or procedure for resolving them; a ritual or procedure that requires the active participation of both patient and therapist and that is believed by both to be the means of restoring the patient's health'. As far as these nonspecific features are concerned, the psychologically oriented therapies practiced in the Western world are no different, according to Frank, than the indigenous healing practices found in preindustrialized societies. It should be noted, however, that all four common elements of Western style

psychotherapies and other healing methods identified by Frank refer to structure, i.e. people and other resources. The healing methods may differ with regard to the two other dimensions of quality of care identified by Donabedian [45], namely process, i.e. the activities of providing care which utilize resources and produce outcomes (what is being done and how it is being done,) and outcome, i.e. the result of the clinical intervention as portrayed by the patient's health status and quality of life. For this reason, the word 'psychotherapy' should be reserved for the type of activity described in Frank's definition, while Tseng's broader concepts should be saved for all healing methods including those in which the effectiveness and quality of care has not yet been demonstrated.

In terms of the theory of demoralization outlined above, psychotherapy is effective by separating distress from subjective incompetence, by attempting to relieve distress or subjective incompetence, or both. This is achieved through attempts to prevent or relieve perceived stress, increase social support, or raise the patient's self-esteem. While relief or prevention of demoralization is the immediate goal of psychotherapy, some modalities go beyond this goal and aim at increasing the patient's resilience (the opposite of subjective incompetence) and restoring a sense of coherence and harmony in the patient's self [46].

Faced with a set of clinical manifestations that might require psychotherapy in a person from a different culture, a psychotherapist would have to first identify the 'assumptive world', i.e. the tacit knowledge shared by the patient and the clinician. This includes values, value orientations and sentiments of the patient, and requires a reconstruction of the latter's personal and collective *Umwelten* and, possibly, a revision of the clinician's own *Umwelten*. The need for a thorough understanding of the *Umwelt* was recognized by Spero Manson during his research on American Indians; this author reached the conclusion that the recognition of depression in this group requires not only a study of the symptoms but also 'the social contexts and cultural forces that shape one's everyday world, that give meaning to interpersonal relationships and life events' [47]. At least some of the subjects studied by Manson might have been demoralized and not depressed, i.e. willing but unable to get out of their predicament.

Next, the psychotherapist would have to determine if demoralization is present, study its sources and arrive at a treatment plan. The study of demoralization requires a thorough understanding of the idioms of distress and subjective incompetence [39]. At this point it is important to determine if the patient is just distressed or also experiencing subjective incompetence (i.e. if the patient is demoralized). If demoralized, the stage of demoralization would have to be ascertained by assessing if the subjective incompetence has evolved into its more severe forms, helplessness, hopelessness, and suicidal ideation, intent and plan.

Although demoralization cuts across both psychiatric and non-psychiatric diagnoses, its clinical significance depends on a number of factors. (a) The clinical context of its appearance: Is demoralization a risk factor, a prodromal phase of a mental disorder, or a trigger for exacerbation or recurrence of psychiatric distress symptoms?

(b) Patient's perception of the intensity of the stress: How stressful is the situation as perceived by the patient? (c) Patient's perception of availability and adequacy of social support.

Given the methodological challenges reviewed above, the variability in the life stories of the patients and the varying and ever changing impact of culture in the pathogenesis of mental disorders, the path from clinical presentation to demoralization and to a psychiatric diagnosis in a cross-cultural context can be complicated and difficult. This is largely due to the limitations of our current diagnostic systems. In moving from the clinical presentation to the diagnostic end point and selecting a treatment modality, cultural psychotherapists might consider using a combination of two approaches: the 'clinimetrics' approach, introduced in medicine by Feinstein [42] and advocated for psychiatry by Fava [43], and the 'perspectival' or 'perspectivistic' approach, proposed by McHugh and Slavney, [48]. Clinimetrics refers to the measurement of areas included in clinical reasoning but not covered by diagnostic taxonomy, such as staging of the disease, severity of the comorbidity, perceived stress, social supports, resilience, and previous response to treatment [46, 47]. Several systems for the staging of mental disorders are already available and their cross-cultural application needs to be investigated [47].

Once the clinical data have been organized in this fashion, the next step would be to determine the best perspective or combination of perspectives that enable the most parsimonious and comprehensive explanation of the clinical data on the basis of the scientific evidence available. McHugh and Slavney [48] identified four perspectives for the interpretation of clinical data in psychiatry: diseases, dimensions, behaviors and life stories. The combined use of these approaches would allow the individualization of the treatment strategy, establishment of incremental validity of the clinical judgment and adaptation to the context of the problem as it evolves. In short, this process will allow the cultural psychiatrist or psychotherapist to move from clinical data to clinical facts. It will also allow the appropriate selection of interventions (treatment modalities), of which psychotherapy would be an essential option, but not necessarily the only option.

The various healing methods may be classified according to their theoretical orientation and postulated locus of intervention in the biopsychosocio-cultural and spiritual spectrum. For example, meditation and yoga derive their rationale from biological or bio-psychological explanations; psychoanalysis and other psychodynamic therapies, client-centered therapy, cognitive, behavioral and cognitive-behavioral therapies are based on psychological formulations; marital, family, interpersonal and group therapies are grounded in the social sciences; and some, but not all, of the so-called 'culture-embedded practices' are inspired by religious, spiritual, and cosmocentric or metaphysical principles. While many of these modalities attempt to reverse pathology, other modalities, such as well-being therapy and positive psychotherapy, capitalize on the patient's strengths. Combined techniques may be used; for example, laying hands or massage may be combined with prayer or meditation, a concept emulated in many modern wellness centers. The focus of therapy may shift from spiritual, symbolic and abstract to sensory and concrete. As Koss-Chioino [49] noted, spiritual interventions allow the healer to raise the hope of a cure by converting a dyad into a triad. The interaction among a spiritual power, the healer and the patient makes the management of the therapeutic relationship much more flexible by expanding the possibilities.

Cultural Considerations

In recent years, detailed and elegant cross-cultural studies have been conducted on issues related to finding the appropriate modality, overcoming communication obstacles, examining the effectiveness of Western-style psychotherapies in non-Western cultures, and designing appropriate models for interventions [43, 50–53]. Clinically relevant research has been conducted on all four elements of psychotherapy identified by Frank, and only a brief thematic sketch can be given here.

The first element is the relationship between the demoralized person and the psychotherapist. It has been well recognized that a thorough understanding of the patient's cultural background is essential to establish a therapeutic alliance, particularly at the beginning of therapy. A related issue is the match of a psychotherapeutic modality not only with the patient's presenting psychopathology and personality profile but also, and most importantly, with his or her ethnic and cultural background. Cultural sensitivity, knowledge, empathy and insight have been identified as additional qualities a cultural psychotherapist must have beyond competence, concern and experience [2, pp. 590–591]. In both Western and non-Western cultures, the psychotherapist has a catalytic effect on the patient. Non-Western cultures place greater reliance on altered states of consciousness to elicit the catalytic effect. Such states are probably experienced as an embrace of the universe and supported by a perceived sense of freedom from the constraints of time, space and logic.

The second element is the setting for the healing. Societal negative attitudes towards any type of deviant behavior construed as mental disorder may detract patients from coming to treatment, participating in the healing process, and adhering to the therapist's suggestions and recommendations. In general, the more culturally friendly the setting is, the more successful the intervention will be.

The third element is a rationale leading to a ritual or a procedure. The foundation on a theory of mind and human behavior distinguishes psychotherapy from informal counseling and advice. The need for appropriate adjustments in theoretical orientations to make them culturally relevant has received considerable attention. This is particularly important in attempts to apply the mainstream modalities of psychotherapy developed in Europe and the United States to other cultures. As Kirmayer [54] states, 'every system of psychotherapy depends on implicit models of the self, which, in turn, are based on cultural concepts of the person'. He goes on to remind us that the cultural concept of the person that underwrites most forms of mainstream psychotherapy is based on Euro-American values of individualism. This is to be contrasted with the sociocentric, ecocentric and cosmocentric views that characterize many other cultures. To this it could be added that, historically, the Cartesian dichotomy of matter and mind never existed or gained ground in certain cultures, i.e. in the great traditions of China and India. An example of an attempt in this direction is the 'Cultural Accommodation Model', proposed by Leong and Lee [55], consisting of three phases: identification of cultural gaps in the existing theory that may affect its cultural validity; selection of culturally relevant constructs and models from the cross-cultural, ethnic and racial minority research to accommodate the existing theory; and examination and analysis of the accommodated theory to assess its incremental validity. If Western-style psychotherapies are planned, for patients unfamiliar with or biased against this type of approach, a suitable preparation is necessary to orient them to the process and guide their expectations if such modalities will be employed.

The fourth element is the ritual or procedure itself. The presenting problem has to be understood in the context of the patient's individual, familial, social and cultural background. Cultural distortions in transference and countertransference have to be recognized and worked out [56]. Culture-sensitive approaches to psychotherapy have been developed, such as the narrative methods for the treatment of the after effects of severe trauma. These methods capitalize on the oral traditions of certain non-Western cultures, having the sufferer assume the role of a witness, rather than a patient [57–60]. As Kleinman [61] noted, narratives allow the healer to pay attention to the patient's perceptions and constructions of the existential struggle and its social context. An understanding of the social context opens up the possibility of public health interventions leading to primary prevention.

Research Prospects

Distressed and demoralized people in non-Western countries and immigrants or refugees in Western countries seek help from a variety of sources: traditional healers, religious leaders, counseling services and professionals trained in the West who may, at times, combine Western methods with traditional medicine (e.g. Ayurvedic and traditional Chinese practices). However, more quantitative studies are needed to evaluate the effectiveness of the different healing methods in use. Several areas of research deserve further exploration such as the effectiveness of culture-embedded or influenced methods, of the combination of those methods with Western procedures, and the provision of Western methods alone.

As stated above, the four elements shared by all healing methods are all structural. Their effectiveness should be evaluated both within and across cultures not only in terms of structure but also with regard to process and outcome [45]. In turn, the methods and scales to assess distress, subjective incompetence, and demoralization were developed and used primarily in the United States, Canada, Italy, Australia, New Zealand and Israel. Their appropriateness and validity in other countries, societies and cultures has to be demonstrated.

Multicultural studies of healing methods should be conducted in which distress and demoralization are studied simultaneously using the same methodological framework in different societies. Such undertakings may not be easy when dealing with culture-embedded practices. Scientific research may be viewed as intrusive in the quasi-religious setting of traditional healing. Controlled studies may be difficult to carry out because traditional healing practices are often informal and short-lived.

The process of psychotherapy could be assessed by using the clinimetrics and 'perspectivistic' approaches mentioned. Also, more studies are needed to deepen our understanding of the impact of cultural factors on the practice of Western-style psychotherapy and the contribution of those factors to the mechanism and outcome of specific therapies. Ideally, the design for research on outcomes should be cluster randomized controlled trials. This type of design demonstrated the effectiveness of group interpersonal psychotherapy for depression in rural Uganda, and of psychosocial interventions led by lay health counselors for depressive and anxiety disorders in primary care in Goa, India [62, 63].

Major inroads have been made in the study of the technical aspects of psychotherapy but more exploration is needed in several areas, including the effectiveness of methods eliciting culturally mediated learning and the inclusion of experienced and respected native healers or lay health counselors in the treatment team.

To conclude, cross-cultural research on demoralization and psychotherapy offers great promise, as shown by the initiatives to include cultural formulation in Western diagnostic systems, the establishment of special curricula on cultural sensitivity for professional training and continuing education, and a renewed interest in the new field of global mental health.

References

1 Pattison EM, Wintrob R: Folk healing: possession and exorcism in contemporary America. J Oper Psychiatr 1981;12:12–30.

2 Tseng W-S: Handbook of Cultural Psychiatry. San Diego, Academic Press, 2001.

3 Griffith EEH, Young J: A cross-cultural introduction to the therapeutic aspects of Christian religious ritual; in Comas-Diaz L, Griffith EEH (eds): Clinical Guidelines in Cross-Cultural Mental Health. New York, John Wiley, 1988, pp 69–89.

4 Frank JD, Frank JB: Persuasion and Healing. A Comparative Study of Psychotherapy. Baltimore, Johns Hopkins University Press, 1991.

5 Leighton AH: My Name Is Legion: Foundations for a Theory of Man in Relation to Culture. New York, Basic Books, 1959.

6 Jaspers K: General Psychopathology. Translated by Hoenig J, Hamilton MW, with an introduction by McHugh PR, vols I and II. Baltimore, Johns Hopkins University Press, 1997.

7 Cassirer E: Philosophie der symbolischen Formen. 1. Die Sprache. Berlin, Bruno Cassirer, 1955. Translated as the Philosophy of Symbolic Forms. 1. Language. New Haven, Yale University Press, 1955.

8 Cassirer E: Philosophie der symbolischen Formen. 2. Das mythische Denken. Berlin, Bruno Cassirer, 1955. Translated as the Philosophy of Symbolic Forms. 2. Mythical Thought. New Haven, Yale University Press, 1955.

9 Cassirer E: Philosophie der symbolischen Formen. 3. Phänomenologie der Erkenntnis. Berlin, Bruno Cassirer, 1957. Translated as The Philosophy of Symbolic Forms. 3. The Phenomenology of Knowledge. New Haven, Yale University Press, 1957.

10 von Uexkull J: Streifzuge durch die Umwelten von Tieren und Menschen, translated as 'A Stroll through the Worlds of Animals and Men: A Picture Book of Invisible Worlds'; in Schiller CH (ed): Instinctive Behavior. The Development of a Modern Concept. New York, International Universities Press, 1957, pp 5–80.

11 de Figueiredo JM: Demoralization and psychotherapy: a tribute to Jerome D. Frank, MD, PhD (1909–2005). Psychother Psychosom 2007;76:129–133.

12 Engel GL: A psychological setting of somatic disease: the 'giving up-given up complex'. Proc R Soc Med 1967;60:553–555.

13 Engel GL: A life setting conducive to illness: the giving up-given up complex. B Menninger Clin 1968; 32:355–365.

14 Caplan G: Principles of Preventive Psychiatry. New York, Basic Books, 1964.

15 Gruenberg EM: The social breakdown syndrome and its prevention; in Caplan G (ed): American Handbook of Psychiatry. New York, Basic Books, 1974, pp 697–711.

16 Kluckhohn CK: Values and value orientations in the theory of action; in Parsons T, Shils EA (eds): Toward a General Theory of Action. Cambridge, Harvard University Press, 1951, p 395.

17 Kluckhohn F, Strodtbeck F: Variations in Value Orientations. New York, Peterson & Row, 1961.

18 Linton R: The Study of Man. An Introduction (student edition). New York, Appleton Century Crofts, 1964.

19 de Figueiredo JM, Frank JD: Subjective incompetence, the clinical hallmark of demoralization. Compr Psychiatry 1982;23:353–363.

20 Lewin K: A Dynamic Theory of Personality. New York, McGraw-Hill, 1935.

21 de Figueiredo JM: Deconstructing demoralization: distress and subjective incompetence in the face of adversity; in Frank J, Alarcon R (eds): The Psychotherapy of Hope: The Legacy of Persuasion and Healing. Baltimore, Johns Hopkins University Press, 2012, pp 107–124.

22 National Comprehensive Cancer Network: Distress management clinical practice guidelines in oncology. JNCCN 2003;1:344–374.

23 Jacobsen P, Donovan K, Trask M, Fleishman S, Zabora J, Baker F, Holland JC: Screening for psychologic distress in ambulatory cancer patients: a multicenter evaluation of the distress thermometer. Cancer 2005; 103:1494–1502.

24 Abramson LY, Metalsky GI, Alloy LB: Hopelessness depression: a theory-based sub-type of depression. Psychol Rev 1989;962:358–372.

25 Dohrenwend BP, Shrout PE, Egri G, Mendelsohn FS: Non-specific psychological distress and other measures for use in the general population. Arch Gen Psychiatry 1980;37:1229–1236.

26 Fabbri S, Fava GA, Sirri L, Wise TN: Development of a New Assessment Strategy in Psychosomatic Medicine: the Diagnostic Criteria for Psychosomatic Research; in Porcelli P, Sonino N (eds): Psychological Factors Affecting Medical Conditions. A New Classification for DSM-V. Adv Psychosom Med. Basel, Karger, 2007, vol 28, pp 1–20.

27 Fava GA, Freyberger HJ, Bech P, Christodoulou G, Sensky T, Theorell T, Wise TN: Diagnostic criteria for use in psychosomatic research. Psychother Psychosom 1995;63:1–8.

28 Stewart JW, Mercier MA, Quitkin FM, McGrath PJ, Nunes E, Young J, Ocepek-Welikson K, Tricamo E: Demoralization predicts nonresponse to cognitive therapy in depressed outpatients. J Cognitive Psychother 1993;7:105–116.

29 Tellegen A, Ben-Porath YS, McNulty JL, Arbisi PA, Graham JR, Kaemmer B: The MMPI-2 Restructured Clinical (RC) Scales: Development, Validation, and Interpretation. Minneapolis, University of Minnesota Press, 2003.

30 Kissane DW, Wein S, Love A, Lee XO, Kee PL, Clarke DM: The Demoralization Scale: a report of its development and preliminary validation. J Palliat Care 2004;20:269–276.

31 Cockram C, Doros G, de Figueiredo JM: Diagnosis and measurement of subjective incompetence, the clinical hallmark of demoralization. Psychother Psychosom 2009;78:342–345.

32 Kisely SR, Shannon P: Demoralization, distress, and pain in older Western Australians. Aust NZ J Publ Heal 1999;23:531–533.

33 Spencer DJ: Anomie and demoralization in transitional cultures: the Australian Aboriginal model. Transcult Psychiatry 2000;37:5–10.

34 Kirmayer L, Simpson C, Cargo M: Healing traditions: culture, community and mental health promotion with Canadian Aboriginal peoples. Austr Psychiatry 2003;11:815–823.

35 Briggs L, MacLeod AD: Demoralization – a useful conceptualization of non-specific psychological distress among refugees attending mental health services. Int J Soc Psychiatry 2006;52:512–524.

36 Briggs L, Talbott TC, Melvin K: An exploratory study of demoralization and migration experience. Int Rev Mod Sociol 2007;33:193–209.

37 Briggs L, MacLeod S: Demoralization or clinical depression? Enhancing understandings of psychological distress in resettled refugees and migrants. WCPRR 2010;5:86–98.

38 de Figueiredo JM: Depression and demoralization: phenomenological differences and research perspectives. Compr Psychiatry 1993;34:308–311.

39 Nichter M: Idioms of distress: alternatives in the expression of psychosocial distress. Cult Med Psychiatry 1981;5:379–408.

40 Kleinman A: Culture, depression and the 'new' cross-cultural psychiatry. Soc Sci Med 1977;11:3–11.

41 Kessler RC, McGonagle KA, Zhao S, Nelson CB, Hughes M, Eshelman MA, Wittchen H-C, Kendler KS: Lifetime and 12 month prevalence of DSM-III-R psychiatric disorder in the United States. Results from the National Comorbidity Survey. Arch Gen Psychiatry 1994;51:8–19.

42 Feinstein AR: Clinical Judgment. Baltimore, Williams & Wilkins, 1967.

43 Fava GA, Rafanelli C, Tomba E: The clinical process in psychiatry: a clinimetric approach. J Clin Psychiatry 2012;73:177–184.

44 Tseng W-S: Culture and psychotherapy. Review and practical guidelines. Transcult Psychiatry 1999;36: 131–179.

45 Donabedian A: Evaluating the quality of medical care. Milbank Q 1966;44:166–203.

46 Mishne J: Multiculturalism and the Therapeutic Process. New York, Guilford Press, 2002.

47 Manson SM: Culture and major depression: current challenges in the diagnosis of mood disorders. Psychiatr Clin N America 1995;18:487–501.

48 McHugh PR, Slavney PR: The Perspectives of Psychiatry, ed 2. Baltimore, Johns Hopkins University Press, 1998.

49 Koss-Chioino JD: the experience of spirits: ritual healing as transactions of emotions (Puerto Rico); in Andritzky W (ed): Yearbook of Cross-cultural Medicine and Psychotherapy: Ethno-Psychotherapy. Berlin, Verlag für Wissenschaft und Bildung, 1996.

50 Okpaku S (ed): Clinical Methods in Transcultural Psychiatry. Washington, American Psychiatric Press, 1998.

51 Tseng W-S, Chang SC, Nishizono M (eds): Asian Culture and Psychotherapy: Implications for East and West. Honolulu, University of Hawaii, 2005.

52 Berzoff J, Glanagan LM, Hertz P (eds): Inside Out and Outside In. Psychodynamic Clinical Theory and Psychopathology in Contemporary Multicultural Contexts, ed 2. Lanham, Jason Aronson, 2007.

53 Negy C (ed): Cross-Cultural Psychotherapy: Toward a Critical Understanding of Diverse Clients, ed 2. Reno, Bent Tress Press, 2008.

54 Kirmayer LJ: Psychotherapy and the cultural concept of the person. Transcult Psychiatry 2007;44: 232–257.

55 Leong FTL, Lee S-H: A Cultural Accommodation Model for cross-cultural psychotherapy: illustrated with the case of Asian-Americans. Psychother Theor Res Pract Train 2006;43:410–423.

56 Comas-Diaz L, Jacobsen FM: Ethnocultural transference and counter-transference in the therapeutic dyad. Am J Orthopsychiatry 1991;61:392–406.

57 Cienfuegos AJ, Monelli C: The testimony of political repression as a therapeutifc instrument. Am J Orthopsychiatry 1983;53:43–51.

58 Igreja V, Kleijn WC, BJ, Van Dijk JA, Verschuur M: Testimony method to ameliorate post-traumatic stress symptoms. Community-based intervention study with Mozambican civil war survivors. Br J Psychiatry 2004;184:251–257.

59 Onyut LP, Neuner F, Schauer E, Ertl V, Odenwald M, Schauer M, Elbert T: Narrative Exposure Therapy as a treatment for child war survivors with posttraumatic stress disorder: two case reports and a pilot study in an African refugee settlement. MBC Psychiatry 2005;5:7.

60 Luebben S: Testimony work with Bosnian refugees: living in legal limbo. Br J Guid Couns 2003;31:393–402.

61 Kleinman A: The Illness Narratives: Suffering, Healing, and the Human Condition. New York, Basic Books, 1988.

62 Bass J, Neugebauer R, Cloagherty KF, Verdell H, Vickramaratne P, Ndogoni L, Speelaran L, Weissman M, Bolton P: Group interpersonal psychotherapy for depression in rural Uganda: 6 month outcomes randomized controlled trial. Br J Psychiatry 2006;188:567–573.

63 Patel V, Weiss HA, Chowdhary N, Naik S, Pednekar S, Chatterjee S, De Silva M J, Bhat B, Araya R, King M, Simon G, Verdeli H, Kirkwood BR: Effectiveness of an intervention led by lay health counselors for depressive and anxiety disorders in primary care in Goa, India (MANAS): a cluster randomized controlled trial. Lancet 2010;376:2086–2095.

John M. de Figueiredo, MD, ScD
Department of Psychiatry
300 George St., Suite 901
New Haven, CT 06511 (USA)
E-Mail john.defigueiredo@yale.edu

Alarcón RD (ed): Cultural Psychiatry.
Adv Psychosom Med. Basel, Karger, 2013, vol 33, pp 88–96 (DOI: 10.1159/000348741)

Ethnopsychopharmacology and Pharmacogenomics

Hernán Silva

Faculty of Medicine, University of Chile and Biomedical Neuroscience Institute (BNI), Santiago, Chile

Abstract

Significant differences in response to psychotropic drugs are observed in various ethnic and cultural groups. Ethnopsychiatry is the study of how culture and genetic differences in human groups determine and influence the response to psychotropic agents. Meanwhile, pharmacogenomics studies the influence of genetic variations in the response of patients to different drugs. Pharmacogenetic tests are used to predict drug response and the potential for adverse effects. There are important genetic variations that influence the metabolism and action of psychotropic drugs in different ethnic groups. As examples, the frequencies of CYP2D6 polymorphisms and of the long and short alleles of the promoter region of the serotonin transporter are analyzed. Studies found significant differences in the frequency of polymorphisms of both genes in different countries and ethnic groups. On the basis of this review, the importance of considering ethnic and cultural factors in the prescription of drugs and in the need of further pharmacogenetic studies in different countries and geographical regions is reaffirmed.

Copyright © 2013 S. Karger AG, Basel

The assumption of universality in the ways psychiatric medications are prescribed and experienced is very common. This view, however, conveys the misconception that ethnic and cultural factors on pharmacotherapeutic responses are negligible. This may be partly based on the fact that the majority of the psychopharmacological drugs have been developed and tested in North America and Western Europe, where the experimental population samples included an overwhelming majority of Caucasian men and women [1]. Yet, significant differences in response to psychotropics drugs have been observed in different ethnic groups. For example, Asian inpatients appear to require lower doses of haloperidol and neuroleptics in general in comparison with their Caucasian counterparts. At equivalent doses, Asian schizophrenic patients and Asian normal controls exhibit plasma haloperidol concentrations 50% greater than

Caucasian, and also have higher plasma prolactin levels [1]. These observations suggest the presence of pharmacokinetic and pharmacodynamic differences that would explain why Asian individuals require lower doses of neuroleptics to achieve similar therapeutic responses.

Ethnopsychopharmacology has been defined as the study of how culture and genetic differences of natural social groupings determine and influence response to psychotropic medications [2]. This discipline recognizes variance in the frequency of genetic polymorphisms across populations, taking into consideration the numerous exogenous factors that impact or alter pharmacological efficacy. It also emphasizes the importance of culture's impact on the biological efficacy of psychiatric medications. Cultural variations in diet, as well as the ingestion of other substances together with the presence of certain genetic polymorphisms, impact on pharmacological efficacy. Complementary or alternative forms of treatment (with medical herbs for example), and the great variability in how culture influences the perception of the therapeutic and adverse effects of medications as well as the placebo effect are all additional powerful factors in this aspect of clinical practice [3].

Psychiatric Pharmacogenomics

Not all individuals respond in the same way to the same medications and these differences are still poorly explained. There are few indicators available to predict the efficacy of psychotropic drugs for any given individual patient. Accordingly, the practice of psychopharmacology is grounded instead on a trial-and-error paradigm. The pattern of drug therapy use in an individual patient is mostly characterized by multiple previous attempts to find the 'right' drug for him or her [2].

Psychiatric pharmacogenomics studies how genetic variations influence the response of a patient to treatment with psychotropic medications [4]. This discipline investigates the ways in which inherited genetic variability impacts psychotropic metabolism and neurotransmitter receptor sensitivity. There are two main applications of current clinical pharmacogenomics, based on the many existing prescription approaches: safety and efficacy [2, 4, 5]. Safety pharmacogenomics identifies genetics polymorphisms affecting the patient's experience of adverse and side effects, using this information to direct drug selection and guide therapeutic dosing. Thd objective of efficacy pharmacogenomics is to use genetic testing to identify specific psychotropics with a high probability of being effective for an individual patient.

The study of pharmacogenetics has been arbitrarily divided into drug disposition and drug targets. Sequence variations in drug-disposition genes can alter the pharmacokinetics of a drug, while those in drug-target genes can change its pharmacodynamics [6]. On the other hand, the pharmacokinetics of a drug includes four stages: absorption, metabolism (transformation), distribution and excretion. If a genetic polymorphism alters the function of a protein involved in the pharmacokinetics of a drug, the concentrations of the parent drug or its active metabolites at the site of the drug's action may also be affected.

The practical application of knowledge in pharmacogenomics has led to the development of tests to predict the likelihood of response and adverse effects with the employment of psychotropic drugs. In 2004 the US Food and Drug Administration (FDA) approved the AmpliChip to genotype the CYP2D6 and CYP2C19 genes. Since, in many academic settings, pharmacogenomic testing has become routinely incorporated into clinical psychiatric practice.

In 2007, the FDA added a black-box warning on the carbamazepine label, recommending testing for the HLA-B*1502 allele in patients with Asian ancestry before initiating carbamazepine therapy because these patients are at high risk of developing carbamazepine-induced Stevens-Johnson syndrome or toxic epidermal necrolysis. This finding has been confirmed in Han Chinese ancestry patients and in other Asian populations, but not in non-Asians in whom HLA-B*1502 is rare [7].

Significant differences have been found in genetic polymorphisms associated with pharmacokinetics and pharmacodynamics in different ethnic groups. The following sections will present findings of studies on two polymorphism widely studied in different ethnic groups.

CYP2D6

The cytochrome P450 family is probably the most widely studied group of drug-metabolizing enzymes. It includes about 20 enzymes involved in the metabolism of approximately 90% of pharmaceuticals in current clinical use. Genetic variations in this enzyme 'superfamily' result in individuals having different metabolizing capacities vis-à-vis the majority of psychotropic medications, as SSRIs, first and second generation antipsychotics, mood stabilizers and anxiolytics [4]. Given the large number of CYP450 alleles, a great number of possible genotypes can result from the various possible pairing of variant alleles on the two human chromosomes. The CYP2D6 gene is localized on chromosome 22q13.1. Over 80 functionally different alleles have been reported for CYP2D6 [8], more than 15 of these encode an inactive or no enzyme at all, while others present gene duplications. One of the reasons for the large research interest on this enzyme is the wide interindividual variation in their activity.

Most studies so far have focused on the role of CYP2D6 in the pharmacokinetics of antidepressant drugs that catalyze hydroxylation reactions. Patients are currently classified into four broad metabolic phenotypes: poor, intermediate, extensive or normal and ultrarapid metabolizers:

(a) A poor metabolizer is defined as an individual who has two completely inactive copies of CYP2D6, or one inactive and one deficient copy. When on standard, evidence-based psychotropic doses, these patients often maintain high levels of the drug

Table 1. Frequency of CYP2D6 alleles by race

Classification	Alleles	Frequency of alleles by race, %		
		Caucasian	African-American	Asian
Normal	*1, *2, *39	70	50	50
Reduced	*10, *17, *29, *41	5	35	45
Nonfunctional	*3, *4, *5, *6	25	15	5

Adapted from Shin et al. [6].

in their blood stream, which can lead to excessive adverse reactions and little or no clinical benefit.

(b) Intermediate metabolizers are individuals with one active copy and one inactive or deficient copy. These patients have higher serum levels of CYP2D6 substrate medications at any given therapeutic dose when compared to individuals with two active copies. This may potentially result in incomplete utilization of psychiatric medication and possible increased adverse events paired with suboptimal therapeutic benefit.

(c) Extensive metabolizers have two fully active copies or one active and one enhanced allele. They are present in the majority of the population and, most likely, reach the desired outcomes in standardized psychopharmaceutical protocols.

(d) Ultrarapid metabolizers are individuals with three or more active copies of CYP2D6. They metabolize certain psychotropics faster than expected, needing higher than average doses. Clinically, this may confer a false appearance of a treatment-resistant psychiatric condition [2].

A number of antidepressants and antipsychotics are metabolized primarily by the 2D6 enzyme: desipramine, doxepine, fluoxetine, nortriptyline, paroxetine, venlafaxine, chlorpromazine, haloperidol, perphenazine, risperidone and thioridazine. Other psychopharmacological drugs that are substantially, but not exclusively metabolized by the 2D6 enzyme are: amitriptyline, bupropion, duloxetine, imipramine, mirtazapine, trazodone, aripiprazole and olanzapine. Otherwise, the D26 enzyme plays a relatively minor role in the metabolic clearance of citalopram, escitalopram, fluvoxamine, sertraline, clozapine, quetiapine and ziprasidone [4]. Because CYP2D6 activity may be different in each allele, the phenotype may be determined by the number of functional, nonfunctional, and reduced-functional alleles carried by the person.

The frequency of CYP2D6 alleles in a given population varies across racial and ethnic groups [4, 6, 9, 10] (table 1). This highlights the clinical utility of using genotyping to guide pharmacological treatments in patient populations of different geographic origin and ancestry. The more than 80 recognized CYP2D6 alleles that inactivate, impair or accelerate its function are, to a large extent, ethnically specific. For example, CYP2D6*4 is the most common inactive allele in European populations with a frequency of approximately 20–25%, but is rarely identified in other ethnic groups. This polymorphism is mainly responsible for the high rate of poor metabolizers (5–9%) among these populations. By contrast, CYP2D6*10 and CYP2D6*17 have been found more often in East Asian and Sub-Saharan African populations, respectively. Both of these alleles are associated with lower enzyme activities and lower metabolism of CYP2D6 substrates. The higher frequency of alleles that encode less effective CYP2D6 in Africans and Asians may explain the lower therapeutic dose ranges of neuroleptics and antidepressants observed in Asians and the lower doses of tricyclic antidepressants needed in African-Americans [1].

Duplications or multiplication of active alleles of CYP2D6 associated with ultra-rapid metabolism of medications, also show significant ethnic differences. The frequency of the ultrarapid metabolizer phenotype is only about 2% in Northern Europeans, but about 30% in Ethiopians [4]. As said above, these patients are likely to fail to respond to usual doses of medications metabolized by CYP2D6, since they typically will not achieve therapeutic levels unless treated with extremely high doses of the same drugs.

In the same manner as CYP2D6, there are important ethnic differences in allelic frequencies of other polymorphisms such as CYP2C19, CYP1A2 and CYP2C9. CYP2C19 is particularly important in the metabolism of citalopram and escitalopram, whereas CYP2C9 operates more with nonpsychiatric pharmacological agents.

Serotonin Transporter Polymorphisms
The serotonin transporter (5-HTT) is the site of action of the widely used reuptake inhibiting antidepressants such as selective serotonin reuptake inhibitors and traditional tricyclic antidepressants. Furthermore, it has been associated with several psychiatric disorders with affective symptomatology (such as bipolar, anxiety, eating and substance abuse disorders), and to a pathological behaviors and personality traits related to anxiety, impulsivity and stress [11]. A polymorphism in the promoter region of the gene encoding 5-HTT (HTTLPR) has been associated with antidepressant response. It is a 44-bp insertion/deletion involving two units in a sequence of sixteen repeated elements and possibly influences serotonin transporter expression, with the long (L) allele associated with a twice basal expression compared to the short (S) allele [12]. Differential transcriptional activity caused by this polymorphism would influence complex traits and diseases, such as affective disorders.

Pharmacogenetic studies suggest that in Caucasian populations the L allele is associated with a better response to antidepressants, although negative findings have also been reported [13]. On the other hand, in Asian populations an association between S allele and better response has been reported. A recent meta-analysis study that analyzed separately Caucasian and Asian populations confirmed this difference [14]. Other ethnicities have not been enough studied to reach any conclusion. It is relevant to remark, however, that the L allele is much less frequent in Asian compared to Western populations (tables 2, 3). In table 2, ethnic differences in the 5-HTTLPR in sev-

Table 2. 5HTTLPR LL, LS and SS genotypes and L and S alleles in different countries

Country, ref.	n	Genotype, %			Allele, %	
		LL	LS	SS	L	S
Croatia [15]	665	38.2	47.5	14.3	62.0	38.0
Germany [16]	228	37.3	44.7	18.0	59.6	40.4
Hungary [17]	151	35.1	45.7	19.2	58.0	42.0
United Kingdom [18]	1.940	33.4	48.7	17.9	57.7	42.3
Spain [19]	83	34.9	44.6	20.5	57.2	42.8
Austria [20]	146	34.9	44.5	20.6	57.2	42.8
Russia: Russians [15]	498	31.3	48.8	19.9	55.7	44.3
Russia: Tatars [15]	380	27.9	44.7	27.4	50.3	49.7
Russia: Bahkirs [15]	261	26.4	46.4	27.2	49.6	50.4
Italy [21]	150	14.0	57.3	28.7	42.7	57.3
PR China [22]	103	13.0	31.0	56.0	28.0	72.0
Korea [23]	252	4.8	40.9	54.4	25.1	74.9
Japan [24]	101	4.0	30.7	65.3	19.3	80.7

Adapted from Noskova et al. [15].

Table 3. 5HTTLPR LL, LS and SS genotypes and L and S alleles in different racial or ethnic groups

Ethnic group	n	Genotype, %				Allele, %		
		LL	LS	SS	XL	L	S	VL+XL
African/African-American	1,193	53	37	9	0	72	27	1
Caucasian	6,415	33	48	19	0	57	43	0
Native American	1,020	12	46	42	0	35	65	0
Korean	890	12	34	54	0	29	71	0
Taiwanese	1,019	8	37	45	8	28	67	4
Chinese	814	6	39	50	5	26	72	2
Japanese	612	4	30	64	2.4	19	80	1

Adapted from Katsuragi et al. [25].

eral European and Asian populations are presented [15]. Table 3 compares the 5-HT-TLPR polymorphisms for specified racial or ethnic groups, including subjects selected of clinical and general populations [25]. The low frequency of L allele in Asians weakens the association between them and the response to antidepressants. Otherwise, additional r genetic variants within the 5-HTT gene or other related genes may represent further stratification factors. A second polymorphism within the L allele (rs25531A/G) may determinate a reduced expression of the gene (Lg allele) comparable with the expression due to the S allele. The studies performed before the detection of this mutation should be re-examined, and future investigations should provide a better understanding of the gene's capabilities [26].

Recent meta-analyses exploring the association between 5-HTLPR and antidepressant response have reported contradictory findings [14, 27]. This underlines the need to consider ethnicity as a confounding – or better, implicating – factor in pharmacogenetic studies. This seems more relevant for 5HTTPR, since very different frequencies of this allele among different populations and the increasing evidence of a different effect of a 5-HTTLPR in Caucasian and Asian populations, have been evinced [14].

In recent years the dichotomous classification of 5-HTTLPR polymorphisms has been questioned. In addition to Lg, two common alleles that are longer than the L variant have been identified [28, 29]. An extra-long allele (XL) was found in both African-American and Japanese samples. A single instance of an allele whose length was between that of L and XL alleles (VL) was also observed in a Japanese sample. Another study in Japan reported two XL variants with 18 and 20 repeats [30]. A third study identified alleles with 19 and 20 repeats in Japanese patients. [31]. Furthermore, using a more detailed genotyping of 5-HTTLPR, four S and six L alleles as well as a few other variants (15-, 19-, 20- and 22-repeats) were identified among Japanese and Caucasian subjects [32]. It is noteworthy that extra-long alleles occur in several samples of persons of African and East Asian origin, but they are not reported in any Caucasian group [28] (table 3). An issue to be explored is how the transcriptional efficiency of the XL allele compares with that of the S and L alleles. Additional research is also needed to identify the functional importance of other alleles of 5-HTTLPR polymorphisms.

One aspect which has been infrequently discussed in the literature is whether the high prevalence of the S allele in Asian populations is associated with higher rates of depression or depressive symptoms in this population [28]. The large differences in how to measure depression in different studies makes it difficult to draw firm conclusions. Nevertheless, two reviews based on a large number of comparable community-based studies suggest generally lower rates of depression in East Asian populations despite being mainly allele S carriers [33, 34]. Several hypotheses have been proposed to account for this paradox. One of them points to the stoicism and resiliency associated with Chinese and other Asian cultures, a feature that pushes individuals to tolerate emotional difficulties rather than seek help. Another hypothesis is that East Asians have a great tendency toward somatization of psychiatric symptoms, in part because they may not view psychiatric symptoms as a sign of illness. Also, presentation of somatic symptoms can also be understood as 'ticket behavior' enhancing symptoms that provide access to care [35]. Somatic symptoms are commonly reported in primary care, and many patients who present initially with somatic symptoms go on to endorse psychological symptoms when asked about them directly. Another explanation is that the strong family and social networks in East Asian societies buffer individuals from the potentially negative impact of stressful events [28]. Along the same lines, it has been argued that in collectivistic cultures such as the East Asians, values of social harmony and support act as buffers to reduce stress and resultant affective disorders even among genetically susceptible populations [36].

Conclusions

The evidence indicates that culture and ethnicity are powerful determinants of an individual's response to psychopharmacotherapy. This is particularly important in the field of pharmacogenomics, considering the significant ethnic differences in genetic polymorphisms related to the action and metabolic modalities followed by psychoactive drugs. Ethnopsychopharmacology represents an important contribution to the discussions surrounding pharmacogenomics by contextualizing pharmaceutical use and considering the cultural patterning of exogenous and nonbiological factors that impact the metabolic status. Since both environmental and ethnic factors can vary across locations, clinical trials could be necessary in each population in order to provide recommendations of the proper doses for each individual in each country [37]. Population-based pharmacogenetic studies are needed in different geographic locations (countries and regions of the world) in order to improve drug safety and efficacy.

References

1 Chen CH, Chen CY, Lin KM: Ethnopsychopharmacology. Int Rev Psychiatry 2008;20:452–459.

2 Ninnemann KM: Variability in the efficacy of psychopharmaceuticals: contributions from pharmacogenomics, ethnopsychopharmacology, and psychological and psychiatric anthropologies. Cult Med Psychiatry 2012;36:10–25.

3 Ng CH, Lin K, Singh BS, Chiu EYK (eds): Ethno-Psychopharmacology. Advances in Current Practice. Cambridge, Cambridge University Press, 2008.

4 Mrazek DA: Psychiatric Pharmacogenomics. Oxford, Oxford University Press, 2010.

5 Roses AD: Pharmacogenetics and Drug Development. The Path to Safer and More Effective Drugs. Nat Rev Genet 2004;5:645–656.

6 Shin J, Kayser SR, Langaee TY: Pharmacogenetics: from discovery to patient care. Am J Health Sist Pharm 2009;66:625–637.

7 McMahon FJ, Insel TR: Pharmacogenomics and personalized medicine in neuropsychiatry. Neuron 2012;74:773–776.

8 Teh LK, Bertilsson L: Pharmacogenomics of CYP2D6: molecular genetics, interethnic differences and clinical importance. Drug Metab Pharmacokinet 2012;27:55–67.

9 Bradford LD: CYP2D6 Allele frequency in European Caucasian, Asians, Africans and their descendants. Pharmacogenomics 2002;3:229–243.

10 Zanger UM, Raimundo S, Eichelbaum M: Cytochrome P450 2D6: overview and update on pharmacology, genetics, biochemistry. Naunyn Schmiedebergs Arch Pharmacol 2004;369:23–37.

11 Serretti A, Calati R, Mandelli L, De Ronchi D: Serotonin transporter gene variants and behavior: a comprehensive review. Curr Drug Targets 2006;7:1659–1669.

12 Heils A, Teufel A, Petri F, Stöber G, Riederer P, Bengel D, Lesch KP: Allelic variation of human serotonin transporter gene expression. J Neurochem 1996;66:2621–2624.

13 Serretti A, Kato M, De Ronchi D, Kinoshita T: Meta-analysis of serotonin transporter gene promoter polymorphism (5-HTTLPR) association with selective serotonin reuptake inhibitor efficacy in depressed patients. Mol Psychiatry 2007;12:247–257.

14 Porcelli S, Fabbri C, Serretti A: Meta-analysis of serotonin transporter gene promoter polymorphism (5-HTTLPR) association with antidepressant efficacy. Eur Neuropsychopharmacol 2012;4:239–258.

15 Noskova T, Pivac N, Nedic G, Kazantseva A, Gaysina D, Faskhutdinova G, Gareeva A, Khalilova Z, Khusnutdinova E, Kovacic DK, Kovacic Z, Jokic M, Seler DM: Ethnic differences in the serotonin transporter polymorphism (5-HTTLPR) in several European populations. Prog Neuropsychopharmacol Biol Psychiatry 2008;32:1735–1759.

16 Lang UE, Bajbouj M, Wernicke C, Rommelspacher H, Danker-Hopfe H, Gallinat J: No association of a functional polymorphism in the serotonin transporter gene promoter and anxiety-related personality traits. Neuropsychobiology 2004;49:182–184.

17 Szekely A, Ronai Z, Nemoda Z, Kolmann G, Gervai J, Sasvari-Szekely M: Human personality dimensions of persistence and harm avoidance associated with DRD4 and 5-HTTLPR polymorphisms. Am J Med Genet B Neuropsychiatr Genet 2004;126B:106–110.

18 Surtees PG, Wainwright NW, Willis-Owen SA, Luben R, Day NE, Flint J: Social adversity, the serotonin transporter (5-HTTLPR) polymorphism and major depressive disorder. Biol Psychiatry 2006;59:224–229.

19 Gutiérrez B, Pintor L, Gastó C, Rosa A, Bertranpetit J, Vieta E, Fañanás L: Variability in the serotonin transporter gene and increased risk for major depression with melancholia. Hum Genet 1998;103:319–322.

20 Willeit M, Praschak-Rieder N, Neumeister A, Zill P, Leisch F, Stastny J, Hilger E, Thierry N, Konstantinidis A, Winkler D, Fuchs K, Sieghart W, Aschauer H, Ackenheil M, Bondy B, Kasper S: A polymorphism (5-HTTLPR) in the serotonin transporter promoter gene is associated with DSM-IV depression subtypes in seasonal affective disorder. Mol Psychiatry 2003; 8:942–946.

21 Nonnis Marzano F, Maldini M, Filonzi L, Lavezzi AM, Parmigiani S, Magnani C, Bevilacqua G, Matturri L: Genes regulating the serotonin metabolic pathway in the brain stem and their role in the etiopathogenesis of the sudden infant death syndrome. Genomics 2008;91:485–491.

22 Li J, Wang Y, Zhou R, Zhang H, Yang L, Wang B, Faraone SB: Association between polymorphisms in serotonin transporter gene and attention deficit hyperactivity disorder in Chinese Han subjects. Am J Med Genet B Neuropsychiatr Genet 2007;144B:14–19.

23 Kim DK, Lim SW, Lee S, Sohn SE, Kim S, Hahn CG, Carroll BJ: Serotonin transporter gene polymorphism and antidepressant response. Neuroreport 2000;11:215–219.

24 Katsuragi S, Kunugi H, Sano A, Tsutsumi T, Isogawa K, Nanko S, Akivoshi J: Association between serotonin transporter gene polymorphism and anxiety-related traits. Biol Psychiatry 1999;45:368–370.

25 Goldman N, Glei DA, Lin Y, Weinstein N: The serotonin transporter polymorphism (5-HTTLPR): allelic variation and links with depressive symptoms. Depress Anxiety 2010;27:260–269.

26 Dong C, Wong ML, Licinio J: Sequence variations of ABCB1, SLC6A2, SLC6A3, SLC6A4, CREB1, CRHR1 and NTRK2: association with major depression and antidepressant response in Mexican-Americans. Mol Psychiatry 2009;14:1105–1118.

27 Taylor MJ, Sen S, Bhagwagar Z: Antidepressant response and the serotonin transporter gene-linked polymorphic region. Biol Psychiatry 2010;68:536–543.

28 Goldman N, Glei DA, Lin Y, Weinstein N: The serotonin transporter polymorphism (5-HTTLPR): allelic variation and links with depressive symptoms. Depress Anxiety 2010;27:260–269.

29 Gelernter J, Kranzler H, Cubells JF: Serotonin transporter protein (SLC6A4) allele and haplotype frequencies and linkage disequilibria in African- and European-American and Japanese populations and in alcohol-dependent subjects. Hum Genet 1997; 101:243–246.

30 Narita N, Narita M, Takashima S, Nakayama M, Nagai T, Okado N: Serotonin transporter gene variation is a risk factor for sudden infant death syndrome in the Japanese population. Pediatrics 2001;107:690–692.

31 Kunugi H, Hattori M, Kato T, Tatsumi M, Sakai T, Sasaki T, Hirose T, Nanko S: Serotonin transporter gene polymorphisms: ethnic difference and possible association with bipolar affective disorder. Mol Psychiatry 1997;2:457–462.

32 Nakamura M, Ueno S, Sano A, Tanabe H: The human serotonin transporter gene linked polymorphism (5-HTTLPR) shows ten novel allelic variants. Mol Psychiatry 2000;5:32–38.

33 Beekman AT, Copeland JR, Prince MJ: Review of community prevalence of depression in later life. Br J Psychiatry 1999;174:307–311.

34 Weissman MM, Bland RC, Canino GJ, Faravelli C, Greenwald S, Hwu HG, Joyce PR, Karam EG, Lee CK, Lellouch J, Lépine JP, Newman SC, Rubio-Stipec M, Wells JE, Wickramaratne PJ, Wittchen H, Yeh EK: Cross-national epidemiology of major depression and bipolar disorder. JAMA 1996;276:293–299.

35 Ryder AG, Chentsova-Dutton YE: Depression in cultural context: 'Chinese somatization', revisited. Psychiatr Clin N Am 2012;35:15–36.

36 Chiao JY, Blizinsky KD: Culture-gene coevolution of individualism-collectivism and the serotonin transporter gene. Proc Biol Sci 2010;277:529–537.

37 Rodeiro I, Remírez-Figueredo D, García-Mesa M, Dorado P, LLerena A, Ceiba FP: Consortium of the Ibero-American network of pharmacogenetics and pharmacogenomics RIBEF: pharmacogenetics in Latin American populations. Regulatory aspects, application to herbal medicine, cardiovascular and psychiatric disorders. Drug Metabol Drug Interact 2012; 27:57–60.

Hernán Silva, MD
Av. La Paz 1003, Recoleta
Santiago (Chile)
E-Mail hsilva@med.uchile.cl

Alarcón RD (ed): Cultural Psychiatry.
Adv Psychosom Med. Basel, Karger, 2013, vol 33, pp 97–114 (DOI: 10.1159/000348742)

Cultural Psychiatry: Research Strategies and Future Directions

Laurence J. Kirmayer[a] · Lauren Ban[b]

[a]Division of Social and Transcultural Psychiatry, McGill University, Montreal, Que, Canada;
[b]University of Melbourne, Melbourne, Vic., Australia

Abstract

This chapter reviews some key aspects of current research in cultural psychiatry and explores future prospects. The first section discusses the multiple meanings of culture in the contemporary world and their relevance for understanding mental health and illness. The next section considers methodological strategies for unpacking the concept of culture and studying the impact of cultural variables, processes and contexts. Multiple methods are needed to address the many different components or dimensions of cultural identity and experience that constitute local worlds, ways of life or systems of knowledge. Quantitative and observational methods of clinical epidemiology and experimental science as well as qualitative ethnographic methods are needed to capture crucial aspects of culture as systems of meaning and practice. Emerging issues in cultural psychiatric research include: cultural variations in illness experience and expression; the situated nature of cognition and emotion; cultural configurations of self and personhood; concepts of mental disorder and mental health literacy; and the prospect of ecosocial models of health and culturally based interventions. The conclusion considers the implications of the emerging perspectives from cultural neuroscience for psychiatric theory and practice.   Copyright © 2013 S. Karger AG, Basel

Cultural psychiatry is concerned with the ways in which psychopathology and healing are shaped by cultural knowledge and practices. Cultural differences between individuals and groups are associated with differences in illness behavior and experience. Recognizing these differences is important to provide equitable and appropriate health care [1] but it also can reveal underlying processes that contribute to mental health and illness [2]. All experience emerges from personal developmental histories and life situations that reflect specific cultural contexts. Understanding the interaction of culture, psychology and biology over time is central to the integrative vision of the biopsychosocial approach.

There is a long association between cultural psychiatry and psychosomatic medicine. This stems in part from the recognition that, across cultures, mental and physical health are closely interrelated if not inseparable. Indeed, the very distinction between mind and body that gives rise to the central conceptual problem of psychosomatic medicine is a consequence of a dualistic ontology that has a long cultural history in Western philosophy and medicine [3]. The fact that this dualism persists in everyday clinical thinking, despite efforts to articulate more integrative and holistic theories, reflects our basic cultural concepts of the person [4].

The ways that culture is conceptualized influence research questions and methodologies. In early psychological and psychiatric research, the term culture was taken as synonymous with ethnocultural group. Later studies began to 'unpack' the notion of culture, defining it in terms of the values, beliefs, and practices associated with an ethnocultural group [5]. This operational definition of culture in terms of traits or aspects allowed researchers to begin to explore how culture influences the manifestations and perceptions of and responses to mental disorder. Attention to specific individual manifestations of culture reveal the heterogeneity among group members, in which some people but not others adhered to certain cultural values and practices.

Thinking about Culture and Mental Health

Culture is not simply the aggregate of individual traits but a more or less coherent system of shared meanings, institutions and practices (i.e. beliefs, attitudes and values) [6–8]. According to this view, culture is a repository of meaningful symbols that structure experience both implicitly and through explicit models. These models are deployed through active processes of signification, meaning-making and self-fashioning by specific actors in concrete situations. Whereas the systems view takes culture to consist of a relatively stable set of knowledge, skills and representations carried by individuals and used across diverse social contexts, the process view insists that culture is not just 'in the head' but 'in the world', embodied in institutions, artefacts, technologies, protocols and practices. A focus on process reveals that culture is often fragmented, fluid and context-specific [9–10]. Social structures and enduring systems of meaning emerge from the actions of individuals in concrete situations.

The system- and practice-oriented views of culture are complementary and both are needed to characterize the impact of culture on mental health. The two perspectives can be integrated in a cultural dynamic view that recognizes that culture endures as well as changes, that culture is both context-general and locally situated, and that individuals' meaning-making activities in specific situations generate collective patterns of meaning that can be interpreted as a globally enduring system [11]. The cultural dynamic view encourages researchers to study how culture and psyche 'make each other up' in processes of mutual constitution. This view allows us to shift from the trait view where culture is treated a cause or independent variable in quasi-experimental designs.

Cultural diversity is an expression of human creativity and reflects our capacity to adapt to diverse ecological niches by adopting different patterns of subsistence and social organization. In terms of individual and social function, culture is the software of the mind, transmitted through interpersonal interaction and participation in social practices and institutions. The brain is the organ of culture, the hardware which cultural experience programs by modifying its microarchitecture, and the long period of neuroplasticity that characterizes human brain development occurs precisely to allow the acquisition of complex cultural knowledge, skills and patterns of habitual behavior [12].

Furthermore, culture produces a variety of identities tied to specific aspects of social life including language, religion, ethnicity, or racialized groups. The significance of these culturally constructed categories for health and illness depends crucially on their social meaning. For example, racial identity in the US is a cultural construction that reflects the history of slavery and current structural forces that maintain systems of demarcation, discrimination and disadvantage [13]. Hence, observed biological effects of race on health, like the increased frequency of high blood pressure among African Americans, can be understood not as a direct consequence of some genetic difference associated with race or skin color, but as a consequence of the social stresses that individuals experience as a result of being labeled 'Black' [14].

Unpacking the received categories of culture, race and ethnicity to go beyond stereotypes requires care in how we use existing labels. Research needs to follow a series of steps to: (1) define cultural groups or contexts with a high degree of detail and specificity; (2) consider what social processes give rise to these definitions; (3) identify specific social/cultural parameters relevant to particular outcomes; (4) attend to individual variation within cultural groups; and (5) consider the cultural assumptions of research theory, hypothesis and design.

The aspects of culture, ethnicity and race that are especially important to psychiatry are those associated with significant differences in mental health, because they involve different exposures to social determinants of health or shape the ways that people adapt to illness, through coping, help-seeking and treatment response. In general, understanding the significance of culture for mental health and illness requires identifying specific knowledge, practices, values, ways of thinking or social positions and predicaments that interact with the mechanisms of psychopathology and adaptation or recovery. For example, the observed high rates of schizophrenia and other psychotic disorders among African-Caribbean migrants to the UK may reflect social adversity and structural violence associated with racism and discrimination [15]. The negative impact of migration can be partially mitigated by living in a neighborhood with people from the same background [16]. This impact of ethnic density can only be understood by linking social processes at the level of urban neighborhoods with psychophysiological processes transduce the everyday challenges of negotiating friendly or hostile social environments into bodily and psychological well-being or stressful wear and tear [17].

The notions of ethnicity, race and culture have undergone constant transformation with changes in migration, ideologies of citizenship and national identity, and new technologies. Over time, new hybrid forms of identity emerge and groups define and assert themselves as distinct communities, introducing new actors and positions into the social world. These are not only new categories or identities but new ways of experiencing belonging and creating communities bound together by ways of life.

While the forces of globalization – including greater mobility, economic exchange and exploitation – have increased cultural homogeneity, they have also allowed the emergence of new hybrid forms of culture [18, 19]. Hence, there is no reason to believe that we will arrive at a global monoculture any time soon. Instead, we are likely to face a complex interplay between larger cultural blocs and a great diversity of smaller cultural groups maintained through networking and electronic media that allow connections and maintain communities despite distance and dispersion.

Methodological Strategies in Cross-Cultural Research

Cultural psychiatry presents unique epistemological, methodological and conceptual challenges. Table 1 lists some key epistemological issues in cultural psychiatric research and corresponding methodological strategies and implications. The risk in any cross-cultural generalization is that, in the effort to apply consistent constructs and measures, we assume meaning equivalence and ignore the lack of fit of our constructs with local reality – a version of what Kleinman [20] has called the 'category fallacy'. Both ethnographic work and efforts to establish external validity can guard against this over-generalization.

The methodological challenges faced by cultural psychiatry include the problems of achieving local validity and making meaningful cross-cultural comparisons.

Culturally valid measures must take into consideration local or 'emic' constructs, including popular illness categories and idioms of distress [21, 22]. A variety of tools are available to elicit idioms of distress in the context of illness narratives [23–25]. Identifying these idioms, constructs and categories involves ethnographic research using participant observation, in-depth interviewing and other qualitative methods to characterize the networks of meaning and modes of interpretation that constitute a cultural system of knowledge and practice [26–28]. This type of research allows the clinician to understand the logic of another culture and can lead to methods of clinical assessment and treatment that make sense to patients and their families and that mobilize resources based on developmental experiences and community contexts.

Staying entirely within the local or 'emic' perspective, however, makes it difficult to compare cultures and recognize commonalities. To enable this comparison, researchers typically use constructs and measures developed in Western (European and Euro-American) settings, which they translate and validate across cultures [29, 30]. Of course, the concepts and tools used in research need not come only from the glo-

Table 1. Research issues, strategies and methods in cultural psychiatry

Issue	Strategies	Methods	Implications
Universality of categories and constructs Existing (predominately Euro-American) categories of health and illness are assumed to be universal (category fallacy).	Identify local symptoms and signs of distress and 'emic' categories. Identify local social, ecological validators to set appropriate thresholds for clinical relevant problems or pathology.	Intercultural dialogue and collaboration. Ethnographic research methods that tap indigenous knowledge and illness experience. Epidemiology using expanded pool of symptoms, alternative criteria, alternative key or core symptoms. Keep anchor points in current nosology to allow for comparison and cumulative knowledge.	Introduction of new categories and criteria. Description of existing categories at the appropriate level of generality. Regrouping of existing categories.
Clinical bias Health problems tend to be seen from perspective of professional mental health services rather than larger pluralistic health care system and other social supports and meaning systems.	Examine prevention, healing and health maintenance in community contexts. Include people who do not seek help and who do not meet diagnostic criteria.	Ethnography. Community epidemiology with locally adapted (emic) measures of distress, symptoms, functional status and outcomes.	Broader eco-systemic view of health care. Potential for working with rather than supplanting indigenous systems. Reduced diagnostic bias or error.
Reification of culture Culture tends to be essentialized as traits and as something held by the 'other'.	Focus on culture of medicine, psychiatry and service institutions. Study role of culture in psychopathological processes, healing and recovery. Recognize culture as dynamic system with its own looping effects.	Ethnographic and qualitative studies of how clinicians' deploy cultural knowledge and assumptions in everyday practice. Diagnostic assessment process and outcome research. Comparative studies of uses of culture in practice.	Integration of culture as intrinsic to clinical practice. Role of cultural processes in pathology, coping, healing and recovery.
Limited evidence base Evidence for treatment efficacy based on study of limited range of interventions with unrepresentative samples.	Insure representative samples of relevant populations. Enlarge pool of interventions and outcomes.	Use samples representative of diversity in clinical and community settings. Development and evaluation of culturally based interventions. Clinical trials of indigenous treatments. Use culturally meaningful definitions and measures of outcome.	Availability of broader range of evidence-based interventions. Reorganization of services to complement indigenous healing and helping resources.

Table 1. Continued

Issue	Strategies	Methods	Implications
Focus on pathology Exclusive focus on illness and pathology rather than health and well-being. Culture viewed mainly as barrier to effective communication and delivery of conventional care.	Inclusion of health, well-being and resilience as dimensions of psychiatric theory as well as clinical assessment and intervention. Study of culture as a resource and source of resilience.	Development of measures of positive mental health and well-being, quality of life and flourishing based on local value systems.	Recognition of sources of health and resilience. Mental health promotion through collaboration with local resources.
Focus on individual Exclusive focus on individual rather than family, community, and environment.	Recognition of larger systems in which social determinants, mediators and outcomes of illness are embedded.	Development of social-ecological models and measures of health and illness. Use of longitudinal process measures to allow dynamical system modeling.	Identify community level interventions that may promote well-being and reduce psychopathology. Uncover unexpected dynamic systemic effects (positive and negative feedback loops, sensitivity to initial conditions, chaos, etc.).

balized West. Local constructs from other traditions can be generalized in ways that allow them to be applied across cultures with the potential to shed new light on universal underlying processes.

A further challenge to cultural psychiatric research arises from the fact that we are self-interpreting beings who readily use the language of psychiatry and psychology to re-describe our experience. In so doing, we bring into existence or reify the very processes or states of affairs we claim simply to describe. The philosopher Ian Hacking [31] has called this circularity the 'looping effect of human kinds' referring explicitly to the ways that new concepts in medicine and psychiatry have been taken up and used to create new kinds of persons and subjectivity. Looping effects are examples of the social construction of experience that demonstrate how psychiatric practice itself can influence illness experience, social response and treatment outcomes [32].

Hysteria provides some of the most clear-cut examples of the plasticity of psychopathological experience. Indeed, Hacking's original examples of looping effects were of dissociative disorders – fugue states in the late 1800s in France [33] and multiple personality disorder in the late 1970s and 80s in the US [34] – but more recently he has pointed to the ways in which new genres of pathography like autobiographical accounts of people with Asperger's syndrome have given rise to new notions of self, gender differences, have looped back into a critique of the diagnostic entity and opened a space to talk about adaptive 'neurodiversity' [35]. Some looping effects are general and cut across diverse forms of pathology while others may be more specific owing to the particular vulnerability or mechanisms of a specific type of psychopathology. Studying these looping effects requires methods of history and social science. A short list of the levels at which diagnostic practice can contribute to looping effects would include: (1) the shaping of symptom and illness experience; (2) symptom attribution and interpretation; (3) modes of symptom expression and reporting in clinical and other social settings; (4) self-coping and help-seeking; (5) the social response to labeling (e.g. stigmatization); (6) the meaning and impact on sense of self, identity and social position of psychopharmaceuticals and other treatments; and (7) the course of illness and recovery [106]. Each of these links in the chain from diagnosis to public health outcome should be considered in relationship to specific forms of psychopathology.

Emerging and Enduring Issues in Cultural Psychiatric Research

Addressing the research agenda for DSM-5, Alarcon and colleagues presented an extensive outline of important topics in research relevant to culture and diagnosis [36]. These included the ways in which culture shapes illness experience, help-seeking and the response to treatment, nosological systems, diagnostic categories, criteria and thresholds, illness course and outcome, and the clinical use and social consequences of psychiatric diagnosis. Central problems in cultural psychiatry that ought to receive attention in future research programs include: (1) defining and measuring forms and levels of vulnerability, distress and disability; (2) defining and measuring well-being, strength, and resilience; (3) defining and measuring social determinants of health; (4) developing and adapting culturally appropriate, safe and effective interventions; and (5) defining and assessing therapeutic process and outcomes. Work in all of these areas should include tracing the impact of psychiatric diagnoses and interventions beyond the clinic to examine their wider social implications.

Cultural Phenomenology and the Nature of Psychiatric Disorders

Current psychiatric diagnostic categories are based on a long Euro-American tradition of describing mental disorders buttressed by several generations of research. Along the way, the categories have become entrenched as the natural way to partition mental disorders. Cultural variations are then seen as minor differences in linguistic description, explanation or symptom expression reflecting local knowledge and idioms of distress. However, while current psychiatric nosology tends to assume that the form of mental disorders reflects underlying neural processes, symptom experience and expression are mediated by cognitive-social interpretive processes that are shaped by culture from their earliest inception [25]. As a result there is no culture-free expression of psychiatric illness based purely on neurophenomenology [2, 37]. All experience is culturally mediated through salient metaphors, narrative templates and modes of discourse. Metaphors may begin as creative attempts to describe experience but become standardized and sedimented in conventional narratives and models of illness that people use to make sense of experience. Hence, we need a cultural phenomenology of illness experience to account for the ways in which people actually experience and express their suffering [38]. In exploring these local modes of expression, we can identify particular ways of construing experience that may foster adaptation or that contribute to functional impairment and distress. This work requires renewed attention to the phenomenology of illness experience with an enlarged or open set of diagnostic constructs.

In addition to the choice of specific symptom clusters to characterize psychiatric disorders, current nosology builds certain assumptions about the course and outcome of disorders into the definitions of disorders. The construction of some disorders as chronic conditions (e.g. schizophrenia) forecloses the question of their relationship to milder, subclinical or self-limited conditions that may have a better prognosis. Even if the most severe forms of mental disorder can be identified across very different cultures, the prototypical cases are far outnumbered by milder conditions that may involve mixtures of symptoms associated with different disorders, and that may not reach the threshold for clinical attention in terms of symptom severity, disability and distress. The links between milder, reactive or situational problems and persistent, profound disturbances of functioning are not well understood and it is possible that social and cultural processes play important roles in the transition from perturbation to chronic disability, or in the other direction from disability to recovery. Research is needed on how the cultural pragmatics of communication shape illness experience, clinical diagnosis, and the course of illness.

Cognition and Emotion as Situated, Embodied and Enacted

There is a growing body of evidence that normal cognition is closely tied both to bodily experience and social interaction. Recent interest in situated and embodied cognition draws from diverse fields including cognitive psychology and anthropology, developmental psychology, robotics and philosophy [39, 40]. This involves a shift in perspective from emphases on mental representations and internal cognitive processes to a view of mental processes as depending on bodily expression or enactment in specific social contexts or situations. Research on embodiment has documented the ways that thoughts, feelings and judgments are affected by bodily states, motivations, and actions [41, 42]. This work can provide a developmental and social history to the emergence and elaboration of culture-specific meanings [43]. Situated cognition has revealed the ways that the body, physical objects and social situations participate in 'cognition', effectively extending cognitive processes out beyond the individual [40, 44].

Multiple lines of research have provided evidence that social contexts fundamentally shape cognitive processes. Seemingly automatic cognitive processes and outcomes that are deeply affected by social contexts include self-esteem [45], self-concept [46, 47], and social stereotypes [48, 49], as well as the operation of memory [50]. All of these studies show that social contexts are among the most important regulators of cognition. These studies of ordinary cognition point the way toward better understanding of how social interactions in family, community and clinical contexts, shape illness cognition and adaptation as well as the dynamics of stigmatization and recovery.

Cultural Constructions of Self and Personhood

There is a substantial body of literature examining the neurobiological, social and cultural construction of the self. At times this conflates different uses of the term 'self' which include: (1) as a 'narrative center of gravity' (e.g. 'I am the center of my narrative account of everyday life experiences as well as my autobiographical stories'); (2) as a locus of intentionality and experience (e.g. 'I encounter the world as an observer with my own distinct perspective and concerns'), and (3) as a locus of agency (e.g. 'I see myself as the initiator of my actions and am present to others as a social actor'). All three of these versions of the self are socially embedded and enacted. As a result, the quality of self-experience varies across cultures.

The self can be thought of in terms of a series of spheres or domains of action and experience from the most private to the most public [51]. The boundaries between self and other vary with cultural configurations of the self. Many people in East Asian societies conceive of the self in more relational or collectivistic terms compared to the emphasis on individual autonomy in the West [52]. Cultural psychology research shows that people in East Asian cultures are just as likely as people in Western cultures to perceive a person as a discrete agent but are more willing to ascribe agency to a collectivity. Hence, for many everyday questions and concerns, the collective is the more relevant boundary of the self.

Consistent with the collectivistic notions of the self, the perspectives of situated cognition and extended mind suggest cognition need not be held in one individual's mind, but instead may be distributed throughout a community in the form of artefacts, institutions, rituals, sites of interaction, and aspects of the social environment. Cultural variation in the self-concept may influence recognition of this distributed nature of mind. While people with an independent self-construal may believe that discrete, physically bounded entities (i.e. a person) are the only kind of system capable of intentional action, people with an interdependent self-construal may form intentions in conjunction with other people so that agency is seen as a property of joint action by the collective.

The contrast between individualistic and collectivistic selves is only one salient dimension of cultural difference. There are cultural worldviews that understand the self as fundamentally embedded in and thinking through the larger, natural environment in what might be called an *ecological* or *ecocentric* self [53, 54]. With the ecological self, cognition is distributed still more widely. Here the self is construed as part of flows or transactions with the environment, which exerts powerful influences on the person's agency or intentionality. This version of self and personhood is found to varying degrees among many indigenous peoples who live close to the land. Similarly, in many traditions, the self may be thought of as deeply connected to or bound up with the activity of an invisible world of spirits or ancestors who must be attended to in making everyday life decisions to maintain the moral order.

Modes of self-depiction, narration or construal depend on how one is situated with respect to others and the social world. Self-construals respond to what the social context holds up as the 'good', 'right' or 'natural' way to be a person. Each person must interpret his or her own context against these shared values. In any given culture, the self may have multiple levels, layers or dimensions, including some notion of a private, interpersonal and ecological self. What varies across cultures may be the extent to which locally elaborated narratives exist centered on each of these aspects, including what counts as a legitimate agent or social actor, and the specific contexts in which the person is expected or enjoined to think in terms of a particular configuration of the self. Psychiatric theory and practice must be enlarged to take into account these different versions of personhood.

Cultural Concepts of Mental Disorder and Psychological Essentialism

Despite efforts to produce clear operational criteria for psychiatric disorders in official nosological systems like the DSM or ICD, most current diagnostic categories are polythetic constructs, with great heterogeneity and fuzzy boundaries. However, the idea of mental disorder possessing clear-cut boundaries in the real world remains intuitively appealing. This appeal can be explained in part through the notion of *psychological essentialism* [55]. According to this notion, people intuitively tend to attribute categories with deep, underlying essences that determine their category membership. This happens in particular with natural kinds (e.g. fruit, animal) as opposed to artefacts (e.g. chair, house), in which people invoke underlying physical attributes that are relatively invariant (e.g. biological structures, genes) when thinking about natural kind categories. Mental disorder tends to be perceived as a natural kind and thus essentialized [56, 57]. Whether or not latent real world constructs possessing deep underlying essences actually exist, the perception that they exist has very real consequences. As such, these processes of perceptions and categorization are an important area of study in their own right.

Whereas the classical approach to categories draws a sharp distinction between concepts and theories, so that the concept identifies the domain that subsequent theories try to explain, the theory-based approach posits that categorization is inextricably linked to explanation [58]. The theory-based model of categorization suggests that cultural theories or meta-narratives may guide attention towards different relevant properties, making certain symptoms more salient than others, i.e. clusters of symptoms may cohere in different ways across cultures. Support for this idea can be found in studies that demonstrate cultural differences in the categorization process such that analytic thinkers (from a Western European cultural background) categorize on a taxonomic basis (i.e. comparing similarity of attributes) and holistic thinkers (from an East Asian cultural background) categorize on a thematic basis (i.e. looking for causal, spatial or temporal relationships) [59, 60].

In categorizing psychopathology, studies suggest that holistic and analytic thinkers weight symptoms differentially (e.g. 'serotonin imbalance', 'lack of family support', 'stressful life event'): holistic thinkers perceive more items as causally relevant, and more 'distal' situational factors as causally central than do analytic thinkers [61]. In keeping with Ahn's [62] Causal Status Hypothesis, which suggests that the categorization of mental disorder is based on the 'deepest' cause perceived, these studies show that differential weighting of symptoms based on holistic and analytic thinking is associated with different criteria by which behavior is pathologized (i.e. found to be abnormal). Culture, thus, suffuses the ways that people recognize and categorize mental disorder.

Global Mental Health, Stigma and Mental Health Literacy

The Global Mental Health movement has pointed out the enormous gap in access to care and mental health outcomes between wealthy and low-income countries. In many parts of the world, people have no access to basic mental health care and people with severe, chronic illness may be treated harshly with physical restraints, confinement and ostracism. To correct these abuses and redress other inequities, leaders have advocated vigorously for the diagnosis and treatment of common and severe mental disorders [63]. Although the global mental health literature often mentions cultural issues, it generally assumes that diagnostic and treatment methods developed in the West can be readily transported to low- and middle-income countries with profoundly different cultural contexts [64]. Confidence in this transportability generally rests on assumptions of biological universality. However, the recent Delphi polling of priorities in research for global mental health puts much emphasis on identifying the impact of culture on effective interventions [65].

Some advocates for Global Mental Health propose using mental health literacy packages in developing countries [66]. The mental health literacy approach targets the public's knowledge and beliefs related to: (a) the ability to recognize specific disorders or different types of psychological distress; (b) risk factors and causes of mental illness; (c) self-help interventions; (d) available professional help; (e) attitudes that facilitate recognition of illness and appropriate help-seeking; and (f) how to seek mental health information [67]. At its core, mental health literacy is concerned with the concordance of lay beliefs with those held by mental health professionals, i.e. getting lay people to identify abnormal behavior correctly using current diagnostic labels (e.g. depression and schizophrenia) through targeted education campaigns.

Medical explanations tend to essentialize mental illness by viewing it as something intrinsic to an individual's biology (brain, genes or other underlying biological systems). Although destigmatization campaigns designed to teach the public an illness model may be beneficial, the available evidence indicates that the biomedical framing of psychiatric illness has not led to wholly positive changes. According to recent studies, the medical model of mental illness may produce another kind of stigma in which the public perceives sufferers as less worthy of blame but more deserving of harsh treatment [68–70]. Read and Harré [71] showed that biomedical explanations produce negative attitudes towards people with mental disorders. The very lack of accountability accompanying the medical model means that suffers may be perceived as dangerous and unpredictable [72]. In an experimental setting, when biological causes of mental illness are emphasized people may endorse harsher, more rejecting attitudes [73].

While some aspects of stigma may be reduced by the medical model, the perceived lack of controllability may actually increase other forms of stigma. In support of this, there is a large body of evidence linking essentialist thinking with prejudice and discrimination [74]. Research shows that symptoms associated with essentialist thinking (e.g. viewed as nonreactive and immutable) are understood in a medicalized way, leading people to desire social distance from sufferers [75]. Other research shows that essentialist thinking about mental disorder is associated with pessimism about recovery and a perception that the sufferer represents a categorically different kind of person [76]. To some extent this may depend on the condition in question and the efficacy of current treatments (i.e. medicalizing has clear costs for schizophrenia) [77].

Different aspects of essentialist thinking may be associated with different kinds of stigma. Some of the negative effects of genetic explanations of mental illness may result from this approach [78, 79]. Knowledge of these links would allow for targeted educational campaigns. It would therefore seem that stigma is not based on moralizing alone and that the medical model is not invariably stigma-reducing, as it can promote essentialist thinking which has the effect of substituting detachment for blame. Research is needed to explore the implications of different models of illness in everyday social contexts for people from diverse cultural backgrounds.

Ecosocial Models of Mental Illness and Wellness

In psychology and psychiatry, the focus on the individual tends to bracket off the environment as an external set of contingencies or social determinants of health. Yet, we are fundamentally social beings and many of the basic mechanisms of cognitive-emotional functioning and adaptation depend on the social environment for their normal development and maintenance. Indeed, recent work in epigenetics makes it clear that the genome itself holds a record of environmental events and its functioning can only be understood in terms of the dynamics of the larger environments with which the genome, cell and individual are in constant transaction [80].

Recognition of this co-construction of the phenotype through gene-environment and brain-environment interactions models of health and illness that go beyond the focus on the individual to characterize social-ecological systems. Interestingly, work with indigenous peoples on local notions of wellness and resilience identifies the importance of levels of strength including family, community and cultural traditions as well as connections to the land [81–83]. Wellness and resilience are expressed through engagement with traditional stories and teachings, relationships across generations, and active participation in culture and community at both local and larger political levels [84]. Psychiatry needs to broaden its models accordingly to thoroughly integrate these social dimensions of well-being and resilience.

Cultural Competence, Safety and Efficacy

Approaches to addressing cultural diversity in mental health services in the US have emphasized the construct of 'cultural competence' which, when operationalized, often amounts to basic instruction in the characteristics of major ethnoracial blocs or, else, ethnic matching of patient and clinician [85–87]. There is limited evidence for the effectiveness of these interventions and much more work is needed to demonstrate how attention to culture and social context makes a difference in clinical practice. The metaphor of cultural competence, which emphasizes clinician knowledge, skills and attitudes, needs to be coupled with attention to the power dynamics of institutions and the over-riding social determinants that affect racialized groups and minorities in society. Work in New Zealand by Maori nurses has proposed the notion of 'cultural safety' as an alternative metaphor to guide culturally appropriate practice by directing attention to issues of power and discrimination in health services and other social institutions [88, 89]. This notion has been taken up by indigenous health researchers, planners and advocates in Canada and extended to provide a general model for improving the quality of health care [90–92]. Research is needed to identify when and how particular models of service and modes of clinical intervention improve access to care, the clinical alliance, and outcomes for specific groups [93].

Cultural diversity raises complex issues in the regulation of pluralistic health care systems. There may be competing claims for efficacy grounded in different epistemologies, with apparently incompatible notions of knowledge and authority [94, 95]. Some of this apparent incompatibility may be resolved by recognizing that different healing systems, based on divergent ontologies, actually target different levels or kinds of outcome. However, recalcitrant problems remain that require further work in bioethics, moral philosophy and social science [96–98]. Attention to culture in mental health services can contribute to building pluralistic civil societies that recognize, protect and preserve the cultural basis of human rights and dignity [99, 100]. As these issues stand at the intersection of health services, social sciences and political theory, interdisciplinary work in this area is needed.

Conclusion: The Future of Cultural Psychiatry

Cultural psychiatry has seen significant advances in recent years with increasing sophistication in theoretical models of psychopathology and a growing body of research. The construct of culture is less a coherent category than a flag planted at the top of a broad hill, claiming conceptual territory that includes a wide range of dimensions of experience. Work in social and cultural neuroscience opens the way to better understanding of the fundamental role of these social dimensions and determinants of mental disorder as well as health and well-being. We have outlined some areas where new conceptual models and methods will allow further progress. However, for cultural psychiatric research to advance, the prevalent forms of neurobiological and genetic reductionism and essentialism must be challenged.

Critical neuroscience, an emerging field at the intersection of anthropology, sociology, philosophy of science and neuroscience can reveal some of the ways in which biological theories in psychiatry are rooted in cultural assumptions [101, 102]. Critical neuroscience locates neuroscience in its current social and historical contexts, exploring the origins, implicit meanings, and limitations of the conceptual metaphors that guide research, theory and practice. In particular, it can identify what gets left out of neuroscientific explanations, particularly the texture of experience and the social and cultural origins, meanings and consequences of brain functions, including the ways we understand the brain [103]. A central concern is with the ways that the findings of neuroscience and the new technologies of brain imaging, genomics, psychopharmacology and brain stimulation influence our sense of self and agency [104–105]. This constructive criticism, a central pillar of cultural psychiatry, can refine the theoretical models and experimental studies at the core of biological psychiatry.

Beyond its concern with social equity and an adequate response to the realities of human diversity, cultural psychiatry can contribute to the core conceptual models and practices of general psychiatry. To realize this potential, research funding, training and the uptake of social science research in clinical practice and policy must all be strengthened. Since the focus on social and cultural issues does not always fit the agendas of profit-making enterprises, an active role by government and other not-for-profit organizations is essential. This poses a direct challenge to universities and other institutions increasingly under pressure to forge partnerships with industry and produce short-term results with demonstrable economic impact. This neoliberal orientation to economic productivity represents a cultural zeitgeist with explicit value choices that may undermine humane and effective psychiatric practice. Understanding the central role of culture in our theories of mental health and illness must, therefore, be central to any vision of the future of psychiatry.

References

1 Alegria M, Atkins M, Farmer E, Slaton E, Stelk W: One size does not fit all: taking diversity, culture and context seriously. Admin Policy Ment Health 2010; 37:48–60.
2 Gone JP, Kirmayer LJ: On the wisdom of considering culture and context in psychopathology; in Millon T, Krueger RF, Simonsen E (eds): Contemporary Directions in Psychopathology: Scientific Foundations of the DSM-V and ICD-11. New York, Guilford, 2010, pp 72–96.
3 Kirmayer LJ: Mind and body as metaphors: hidden values in biomedicine; in Lock M, Gordon D (eds): Biomedicine Examined. Dordrecht, Kluwer, 1988, pp 57–92.
4 Miresco MJ, Kirmayer LJ: The persistence of mind-brain dualism in psychiatric reasoning about clinical scenarios. Am J Psychiatry 2006;163:913–918.
5 Betancourt H, Lopez SR: The study of culture, ethnicity, and race in American psychology. Am Psychologist 1993;48:629–637.
6 Triandis HC: The Analysis of Subjective Culture. Oxford, Wiley-Interscience, 1972.
7 Geertz C: The Interpretation of Cultures. New York, Basic Books, 1973.
8 Rohner RP: Toward a conception of culture for cross-cultural psychology. J Cross-Cultural Psychol 1984;15:111–138.
9 Cole M: Cultural psychology: a once and future discipline. Cambridge, Harvard University Press, 1996.
10 Greenfield PM, Keller H, Fuligni A, Maynard A: Cultural pathways through universal development. Ann Rev Psychol 2003;54:461–490.
11 Kashima Y: Conceptions of culture and person for psychology. J Cross-Cultural Psychol 2000;31:14–32.
12 Wexler BE: Brain and Culture: Neurobiology, Ideology, and Social Change. Cambridge, MIT Press, 2006.

13 Hollinger DA: Postethnic America. Beyond Multiculturalism. New York, Basic Books, 1995.
14 Gravlee CC: How race becomes biology: embodiment of social inequality. Am J Phys Anthropol 2009;139:47–57.
15 Cantor-Graae E: The contribution of social factors to the development of schizophrenia: a review of recent findings. Can J Psychiatry Rev 2007;52:277–286.
16 Shaw RJ, Atkin K, Becares L, Albor CB, Stafford M, Kiernan KE, et al: Impact of ethnic density on adult mental disorders: narrative review. Br J Psychiatry 2012;201:11–19.
17 van Os J: Psychotic experiences: disadvantaged and different from the norm. Br J Psychiatry 2012;201: 258–259.
18 Burke P: Cultural Hybridity. Cambridge, Polity, 2009.
19 Kraidy M: Hybridity, or the Cultural Logic of Globalization. Philadelphia, Temple University Press, 2005.
20 Kleinman A: Anthropology and psychiatry: the role of culture in cross-cultural research on illness. Br J Psychiatry 1987;151:447–454.
21 Kleinman AM: Patients and Healers in the Context of Culture. Berkeley, University of California Press, 1980.
22 Nichter M: Idioms of distress: alternatives in the expression of psychosocial distress: a case study from South India. Culture Med Psychiatry 1981;5:379–408.
23 Weiss M: Explanatory Model Interview Catalogue (EMIC): Framework for comparative study of illness. Transcult Psychiatry 1997;34:235–263.
24 Groleau D, Young A, Kirmayer LJ: The McGill Illness Narrative Interview (MINI): an interview schedule to elicit meanings and modes of reasoning related to illness experience. Transcult Psychiatry 2006;43:671–691.

25 Kirmayer LJ, Bhugra D: Culture and mental illness: social context and explanatory models; in Salloum IM, Mezzich JE (eds): Psychiatric Diagnosis: Patterns and Prospects. New York, Wiley, 2009, pp 29–37.

26 Nichter M: Idioms of distress revisited. Cult Med Psychiatry 2010;34:401–416.

27 Pedersen D, Kienzler H, Gamarra J: Llaki and nakary: idioms of distress and suffering among the highland Quechua in the Peruvian Andes. Cult Med Psychiatry 2010;34:279–300.

28 Lewis-Fernandez R, Gorritz M, Raggio GA, Pelaez C, Chen H, Guarnaccia PJ: Association of trauma-related disorders and dissociation with four idioms of distress among Latino psychiatric outpatients. Cult Med Psychiatry 2010;34:219–243.

29 De Jong JTVM, Van Ommeren M: Toward a culture-informed epidemiology: Combining qualitative and quantitative research in transcultural contexts. Transcult Psychiatry 2002;39:422–433.

30 Van Ommeren M: Validity issues in transcultural epidemiology. Br J Psychiatry 2003;182:376–378.

31 Hacking I: The looping effect of human kinds; in Sperber D, Premack D, Premack AJ (eds): Causal Cognition: A Multidisciplinary Debate. Oxford, Oxford University Press, 1995, pp 351–383.

32 Hacking I: The Social Construction of What? Cambridge, Harvard University Press, 1999.

33 Hacking I: Mad Travelers: Reflections on the Reality of Transient Mental Illnesses. Charlottesville, University Press of Virginia, 1998.

34 Hacking I: Rewriting the Soul. Princeton, Princeton University Press, 1995.

35 Hacking I: Autistic autobiography. Phil Trans R Soc Lond (B) 2009;364:1467–1473.

36 Alarcón RD, Bell CC, Kirmayer LJ, Lin K-H, Ustun TB, Wisner KL: Beyond the funhouse mirrors: Research agenda on culture and psychiatric diagnosis; in Kupfer DJ, First MB, Regier DA (eds): A Research Agenda for DSM-V. Washington, American Psychiatric Press, 2002, pp 219–89.

37 Kirmayer LJ: Nightmares, Neurophenomenology and the Cultural Logic of Trauma. Cult Med Psychiatry 2009;33:323–331.

38 Kirmayer LJ: Culture and the metaphoric mediation of pain. Transcult Psychiatry 2008;45:318–338.

39 Robbins P, Aydede M: The Cambridge Handbook of Situated Cognition. Cambridge, Cambridge University Press, 2009.

40 Rowlands M: The New Science of the Mind: From Extended Mind to Embodied Phenomenology. Cambridge, MIT Press, 2010.

41 Gibbs RW: Embodiment and Cognitive Science. New York, Cambridge University Press, 2006.

42 Barsalou LW: Grounded cognition. Ann Rev Psychol 2008;59:617–645.

43 Kövecses Z: Metaphor in Culture: Universality and Variation. Cambridge, Cambridge University Press, 2005.

44 Menary R: The Extended Mind. Cambridge, MIT Press, 2010.

45 Crocker J: Social stigma and self-esteem: situational construction of self-worth. J Exp Soc Psychol 1999; 35:89–107.

46 McGuire WJ, McGuire CV: Content and process in the experience of self; in Berkowitz L (ed): Advances in Experimental Social Psychology. New York, Academic Press, 1988, pp 97–144.

47 Tice DM: Self-concept change and self-presentation: the looking glass self is also a magnifying glass. J Pers Soc Psychol 1992;63:435–451.

48 Schaller M, Conway LG 3rd: Influence of impression-management goals on the emerging contents of group stereotypes: support for a social-evolutionary process. Pers Soc Psychol Bull 1999;25:819–833.

49 Schaller M, Conway LG 3rd, Tanchuk TL: Selective pressures on the once and future contents of ethnic stereotypes: effects of the communicability of traits. J Pers Soc Psychol 2002;82:861–877.

50 Dodd DH, Brashaw JM: Leading questions and memory: pragmatic constraints. J Verbal Learn Verbal Behav 1980;19:695–704.

51 Hsu FLK: The self in cross-cultural perspective; in Marsella AJ, Devos G, Hsu FLK (eds): Culture and Self: Asian and Western Perspectives. New York, Tavistock Publications, 1985, pp 24–55.

52 Heine SJ: Self as cultural product: an examination of East Asian and North American selves. J Personality 2001;69:881–906.

53 Kirmayer LJ: Psychotherapy and the cultural concept of the person. Transcult Psychiatry 2007;44: 232–257.

54 Kirmayer LJ, Fletcher C, Watt R: Locating the ecocentric self: Inuit concepts of mental health and illness; in Kirmayer LJ, Valaskakis G (eds): Healing Traditions: The Mental Health of Aboriginal Peoples in Canada. Vancouver, University of British Columbia Press, 2008, pp 289–314.

55 Medin D, Ortony A: Psychological essentialism; in Vosniadou S, Ortony A (eds): Similarity and Analogical Reasoning. Cambridge, Cambridge University Press, 1989, pp 179–195.

56 Haslam N, Ernst D: Essentialist beliefs about mental disorders. J Soc Clin Psychol 2002;21:628–644.

57 Haslam N: Psychiatric categories as natural kinds: essentialist thinking about mental disorders. Soc Res 2000;67:1031–1058.

58 Murphy GL, Medin DL: The role of theories in conceptual coherence. Psychol Rev 1985;92:289–316.

59 Nisbett RE: The Geography of Thought: How Asians and Westerners Think Differently – and Why. New York, Free Press, 2003.

60 Ji LJ, Zhang Z, Nisbett RE: Is it culture or is it language? Examination of language effects in cross-cultural research on categorization. J Pers Soc Psychol 2004;87:57–65.

61 Ban L, Kashima Y, Haslam N: Does understanding behavior make it seem normal? Perceptions of abnormality among Euro-Australians and Chinese-Singaporeans. J Cross-Cultural Psychol 2012;43: 286–298.

62 Ahn W: Why are different features central for natural kinds and artifacts? The role of causal status in determining feature centrality. Cognition 1998;69: 135–178.

63 Patel V, Prince M: Global mental health: a new global health field comes of age. JAMA 2010;303:1976–1977.

64 Patel V, Araya R, Chatterjee S, Chisholm D, Cohen A, De Silva M, et al: Treatment and prevention of mental disorders in low-income and middle-income countries. Lancet 2007;370:991–1005.

65 Collins PY, Patel V, Joestl SS, March D, Insel TR, Daar AS, et al: Grand challenges in global mental health. Nature 2011;475:27–30.

66 Patel V, Thornicroft G: Packages of care for mental, neurological, and substance use disorders in low- and middle-income countries: PLoS Medicine Series. PLoS Med 2009;6:e1000160.

67 Jorm AF: Mental health literacy: empowering the community to take action for better mental health. Am Psychol 2012;67:231–243.

68 Farina A, Fisher JD, Getter H, Fischer EH: Some consequences of changing people's views regarding the nature of mental illness. J Abnorm Psychol 1978;87: 272–279.

69 Read J, Law A: The relationship of causal beliefs and contact with users of mental health services to attitudes to the 'mentally ill'. Int J Soc Psychiatry 1999; 45:216–229.

70 Walker I, Read J: The differential effectiveness of psychosocial and biogenetic causal explanations in reducing negative attitudes toward 'mental illness'. Psychiatry 2002;65:313–325.

71 Read J, Harré N: The role of biological and genetic causal beliefs in the stigmatisation of 'mental patients'. J Ment Health 2001;10:223–235.

72 Sarbin TR, Mancuso JC: Failure of a moral enterprise: attitudes of the public toward mental illness. J Consult Clin Psychol 1970;35:159–173.

73 Mehta S, Farina A: Is being 'sick' really better? Effect of the disease view of mental disorder on stigma. J Soc Clin Psychol 1997;16:405–419.

74 Haslam N, Rothschild L, Ernst D: Are essentialist beliefs associated with prejudice? Br J Soc Psychol 2002;41:87–100.

75 Dietrick S, Beck M, Bujantugs B, Kenzine D, Matschinger H, Angermeyer MC: The relationship between public causal beliefs and social distance toward mentally ill people. Aust NZ J Psychiatry 2004;38:348–354.

76 Haslam N, Ban L, Kaufmann A: Lay conceptions of mental disorder: The folk psychiatry model. Aust Psychol 2007;42:129–137.

77 Angermeyer MC, Buyantugs L, Kenzine DV, Matschinger H: Effects of labelling on public attitudes towards people with schizophrenia: are there cultural differences? Acta Psychiatr Scand 2004;109: 420–425.

78 Dar-Nimrod I, Heine SJ: Genetic essentialism: on the deceptive determinism of DNA. Psychol Bull 2011; 137:800–818.

79 Haslam N: Genetic essentialism, neuroessentialism, and stigma: commentary on Dar-Nimrod and Heine (2011). Psychol Bull 2011;137:819–824.

80 Zhang TY, Meaney MJ: Epigenetics and the environmental regulation of the genome and its function. Ann Rev Psychol 2010;61:439–466, C1–3.

81 Fleming JE, Ledogar R: Resilience, an evolving concept: a review of literature relevant to Aboriginal research. Pimatisiwin 2008;6:7–23.

82 Kirmayer LJ, Sedhev M, Whitley R, Dandeneau S, Isaac C: Community resilience: models, metaphors and measures. J Aboriginal Health 2009;7:62–117.

83 Kirmayer LJ, Dandeneau S, Marshall E, Phillips MK, Williamson KJ: Rethinking resilience from indigenous perspectives. Can J Psychiatry Rev 2011;56:84–91.

84 Kirmayer LJ, Dandeneau S, Marshall E, Phillips MK, Williamson KJ: Toward an ecology of stories: Indigenous perspectives on resilience; in Ungar M (ed): The Social Ecology of Resilience. New York, Springer, 2012, pp 399–414.

85 Hernandez M, Nesman T, Mowery D, Acevedo-Polakovich ID, Callejas LM: Cultural competence: a literature review and conceptual model for mental health services. Psychiatr Serv 2009;60:1046–1050.

86 Good M-JD, Willen SS, Hannah SD, Vickery K, Park LT (eds): Shattering Culture: American Medicine Responds to Cultural Diversity. New York, Russell Sage Foundation, 2011.

87 Kirmayer LJ: Rethinking cultural competence. Transcult Psychiatry 2012;49:149–164.

88 Papps E, Ramsden I: Cultural safety in nursing: the New Zealand experience. Int J Qual Health Care 1996;8:491–497.

89 Koptie S, Ramsden I: The public narrative on cultural safety. First Peoples Child Fam Rev 2009;4:30–43.

90 Brascoupé S, Waters C: Cultural safety: exploring the applicability of the concept of cultural safety to Aboriginal health and community wellness. J Aboriginal Health 2009;7:6–40.

91 The Indigenous Physicians Association of Canada: The Royal College of Physicians & Surgeons of Canada. Cultural Safety in Practice: A Curriculum for Family Medicine Residents and Physicians. Winnipeg & Ottawa, IPAC-RCPSC Family Medicine Curriculum Development Working Group, 2009.

92 Smye V, Josewski V, Kendall E: Cultural Safety: An Overview. Ottawa, First Nations, Inuit and Métis Advisory Committee, Mental Health Commission of Canada, 2010.

93 Wendt DC, Gone JP: Rethinking cultural competence: insights from indigenous community treatment settings. Transcult Psychiatry 2012;49:206–222.

94 Gone JP: A community-based treatment for Native American historical trauma: prospects for evidence-based practice. J Consult Clin Psychol 2009;77:751–762.

95 Kirmayer LJ: Cultural competence and evidence-based practice in mental health: epistemic communities and the politics of pluralism. Soc Sci Med 2012;75:249–256.

96 Engelhardt HT Jr: Confronting moral pluralism in posttraditional Western societies: bioethics critically reassessed. J Med Philos 2011;36:243–260.

97 Talisse RB: Pluralism and Liberal Politics. New York, Taylor & Francis, 2012.

98 Talisse RB: Democracy and Moral Conflict. Cambridge, Cambridge University Press, 2009.

99 Kirmayer LJ: Culture and context in human rights. In: Dudley M, Silove D, Gale F, editors. Mental Health and Human Rights: Vision, Praxis and Courage. Oxford, Oxford University Press, 2012, pp 95–112.

100 Kirmayer LJ: Multicultural medicine and the politics of recognition. J Med Philos 2011;36:410–423.

101 Choudhury S, Kirmayer LJ: Cultural neuroscience and psychopathology: prospects for cultural psychiatry. Prog Brain Res 2009;178:261–281.

102 Choudhury S, Nagel SK, Slaby J: Critical neuroscience: linking neuroscience and society through critical practice. BioSocieties 2009;4:61–77.

103 Kirmayer LJ, Gold I: Re-socializing psychiatry: Critical neuroscience and the limits of reductionism; in Choudhury S, Slaby J (eds): Critical Neuroscience: A Handbook of the Social and Cultural Contexts of Neuroscience. Oxford, Blackwell, 2012.

104 Jenkins JH: Pharmaceutical self: the global shaping of experience in an age of psychopharmacology. Santa Fe, School for Advanced Research Press, 2010.

105 Choudhury S, Slaby J: Critical Neuroscience. A Handbook of the Social and Cultural Contexts of Neuroscience. Oxford, Wiley-Blackwell, 2011.

106 Kirmayer LJ, Sartorius N: Cultural models and somatic syndromes. Psychosom Med 2007;69:832–840.

Laurence J. Kirmayer
4333 Cote Ste Catherine Rd.
Montreal, Quebec H3T 1E4 (Canada)
E-Mail laurence.kirmayer@mcgill.ca

Alarcón RD (ed): Cultural Psychiatry.
Adv Psychosom Med. Basel, Karger, 2013, vol 33, pp 115–122 (DOI: 10.1159/000348807)

Bioethical Dimensions of Cultural Psychosomatics: The Need for an Ethical Research Approach[1]

Fernando Lolas

Department of Psychiatry, University Hospital, Interdisciplinary Center for Bioethics, University of Chile, Santiago, Chile

Abstract

Contemporary psychosomatics is a research-based technical discipline and its social power depends on how scientific knowledge is obtained and applied in practice, considering cultural contexts. This article presents the view that the dialogical principles on which bioethical discourse is based are more inclusive than professional ethics and philosophical reflection. The distinction is advanced between rule-guided behavior and norm-justifiable acts (substantiation and justification). The practical implications of good practices in the generation of valid, reliable, generalizable and applicable knowledge are emphasized. For practitioners and researchers, the need to reflect on the distinction between patient and research participant can avoid the therapeutic misunderstanding, a form of abuse of the doctor-patient relationship. In addition, in resource-poor settings, the dilemma presented by the know-do gap (inapplicability of research results due to financial or social constraints) is part of the ethics' realm of the profession. Future prospects include a wider use of research results in practice, but avoidance of the know-do gap (the disparity between what is known and what can be done, particularly in settings with limited resources) requires a synthetic and holistic approach to medical ethics, combining moral reflection, theoretical analysis and empirical data.

Psychosomatics and Behavioral Science as Research-Based Knowledge

At no other time in its history has psychiatry been more dependent on scientific knowledge than it is today. The same considerations apply to related subareas like biopsychosocial medicine, psychosomatic theorization, and psychological medicine in general. Scientific rationality prevails in the construction and application of clinical

[1] During the preparation of this paper, the author received support from the Alexander von Humboldt Foundation (Humboldt Alumni Preis) and from grant R25 TW6056–8 NIH-Fogarty.

guidelines, policy formulation, and delivery of services. Since science is not just a static and fixed collection of facts but a continuously changing flux of data and information, research is the cornerstone of scientific practice in Western societies. Research is a complex social process patterned after the cultural and value-based features of the societies in which it is performed. It aims at the social production and dissemination of valid, reliable, and generalizable knowledge [1, 2]. Its stakeholders are numerous: sponsors, scientists, subjects (or participants) and policymakers. The acceptance and further use of research results is based on the distinction between data and belief. Only information collected under certain conditions and with methods approved by the scientific community count as data useful for the construction of applicable knowledge. Other sources of certainty, like intuition and empathic revelation, are deemed components of the system of certainties but do not enjoy the same status as knowledge constructed by publicly accepted and falsifiable methods. Training of psychiatrists, although emphasizing the role of interpersonal and personality factors, stresses scientific and intellectual proficiency [3].

Scientific research in psychosomatics can be devoted to contextual and organismic factors relevant to mentation, affect and behavior. Among the contextual factors, those related to environment and social aspects are the most relevant. Organismic factors refer to verbal and nonverbal data. The latter include motor behavior and physiological/biochemical information, gathered according to appropriate methodology. Psychiatry and its related disciplines, concerned with mental and bodily health and their disorders at the individual and societal levels, extend beyond medicine. They can be construed as specialized professions based on scientific research and devoted to human welfare [4]. They are concerned not only with healing and curing but also with human enhancement and development of human potentials.

Psychosomatic research can be approached from two points of view: the methodological or epistemological, on the one side, and the ontological or metaphysical on the other. Although this distinction is more of a theoretical nature, it can be said that in both approaches ethical considerations are paramount. It is relevant to stress the fact that ethical reflection is always local, deeply anchored in culture and tradition.

Bioethics, Neuroethics and Applied Ethics

For the practice of a research-based, culture-fair psychosomatics, the most relevant issues are not only *what* to investigate and to *which purpose* but *how* knowledge can be obtained and applied respecting fundamental human values and the dignity of persons in research and healthcare [5]. These considerations extend to the humane use of laboratory animals for obtaining data [6]. The ethics of research has become essential in diagnosis, development of services, improvement of clinical care, and priority setting [7].

Ethics can be understood as that part of philosophy dealing with virtues and duties. It treats human behavior according to an accepted criterion of the good and the appropriate or right. Ethics as value theory is concerned with an evaluation of human conduct in diverse contexts, [8] and it may be considered, on the one hand, a structural condition of human beings and, on the other, a particular set of beliefs on how the good life may be achieved. Rather than descriptive, ethical theorization is prescriptive about what should be done under every life circumstance.

Bioethics emerged in the 20th century after the realization that ends do not justify the means in scientific research if human dignity or fundamental rights are violated, even invoking the welfare of humankind [9, 10, 11]. Flagrant violations were evident in civilized countries. The political abuse of psychiatric practice and research was observed in different contexts. Examples provided by Nazi Germany and Communist Soviet Union need no emphasis [12, 13]. The failure of traditional philosophical reflection for preventing abuse was evident after WWII, leading to the realization that the appropriate form of ethical thinking is dialogical. This implies that any value to implement, any rule to follow or any norm to guide behavior should be legitimized by the consensual elaboration of harms, risks, and benefits beyond private or religious convictions and, at the same time, harmonized with adequate interpretation of the expectations, needs and demands of people with different beliefs. This 'dialogical turn' in ethical reflection marks the emergence of a new discourse. It does not represent a new brand of professional ethics, nor is it a revival of philosophical speculation [14]. It manifests itself in institutions embodying the ideal of dialogue, like committees and commissions at different levels of the social organization (institutional, geographic, and national), formed by people with different backgrounds, interests and positions in a knowledge-generating social system. The voice of lay people is to be heard in all and every form of intervention in mind and body, as asserted by the 1978 Belmont Report, prepared under the sponsorship of the US Government. It expanded and complemented the Nürnberg Code (1947) and the Declaration of Helsinki (1964), landmark documents written in response to a growing demand for reliable orientation in matters concerning the relationship between rights, knowledge, and social power of states, professions, and communities.

The history of philosophical thought shows that the distinction between facts and values has been important in the development of empirical knowledge. Between the value objectivism of Platonic idealism and the subjectivist emphasis of existentialism, the form best representing the dialogical turn and the emergence of bioethics is *value constructivism* [15, 16]. Scientific advances are informed by values and, in turn, influence values according to rules and procedures that have to be established, justified, and accepted, by the people affected by them. Formulation, justification, and application of principles (considered as *prima facie* deployments of value judgments in everyday situations) become essential tools for the work in ethics committees, ethics counseling, and ethics education.

A further consideration should be added in relation to the source of ethical intuition. For some authors, all ethics are equal, and psychiatric ethics is just an application of general rules of conduct to a particular domain. This generalist and philosophical approach contrasts sharply with the idea that each field of enquiry, faced with its particular challenges, should develop ethical procedures following a bottom-up strategy. Thus, problems encountered by psychiatric research are best understood by people who face them in real life situations, and not by imposing a philosophical persuasion upon the behavior of researchers and practitioners. Psychiatric ethics is not ethics applied to psychiatry but ethics in a particular context, one of dialogue and consensual analysis [17], informed by scientific facts and societal constraints.

A special form of bioethics, termed Neuroethics, involves two types of questions: the neural basis of feeling, emotion, and morals as evinced by neuroscientific research, and the social implications of the possibilities opened up by this research, like drug interventions for enhancing mental capabilities or improving performance. Neuroethics, as the confluence of both the analysis of how ethics is based on brain physiology and how neuroscientific discoveries affect society, is particularly relevant to psychiatry and psychosomatics, especially when dealing with methods for diagnosing disorders or therapies involving direct interventions on the central nervous system [18–22].

The dialogical nature of bioethics has made the committee a requisite social institution for the evaluation of practices in healthcare and health research. There are hospital committees, concerned with clinical practice, research ethics committees (sometimes called 'institutional review boards', IRBs), and professional ethics committees. Each of them has its own dynamics and purposes but deliberation is the cornerstone of ethical decision-making in such bodies. It can be said that personal convictions of the members of a committee are confronted with the consequences of their decisions and that in this sense the work of a committee is a mixture between ethics of duties (deontology) and ethics of responsibility (teleology, ethics of goals), and includes, therefore, deontological and teleological stages or phases [23, 24].

In analyzing the importance and impact of new therapies, in applying novel ideas or information, in planning and performing clinical trials, researchers and practitioners alike should consider the context in which work is performed, the aims it envisions, the feasibility of its accomplishment, and the legitimacy of the procedures employed – the essence of Applied Ethics. This applies both to data-gathering activities, to data-organizing ones, and to the application of new knowledge to social needs. In professional practice, the need to consider personal beliefs and moral conscience adds to the complexity of psychiatric bioethics.

Rule-Guided Behavior and Norm-Justifiable Acts

Justification of norms of conduct should not be confused with establishing the fundamental basis of a decision [25]. The latter is typical of technical thinking, in which rules dictate the art. The former is a way of legitimizing actions by a code of conduct. It depends upon communication between persons in a society of equals albeit differing in knowledge and moral certitudes. The tension between these two modes of legitimizing action leads to misunderstandings [26]. Some people believe that moral norms are like physical laws that apply in all and every situation in which technical expertise is demanded. This is a new version of the 'naturalistic fallacy', which equates judgments based on empirical fact or observation with judgments based on moral imperatives. Although the importance of empirical data for value judgments is undeniable, these judgments are not only dependent on what is the case but more on what ought to be according to general beliefs about human nature. The dialogical principle in bioethics is a good reminder that all decisions are based on a 'reflective equilibrium' between a norm and the reality it encounters. A blind application of truths is as damaging as a complete lack of guidance. The dialogical principle extends not only to interactions between persons but also to the confrontation of beliefs and facts. Moreover, any reflection on ethics must consider the issue of power when dealing with the application of knowledge to human affairs. In some areas of the world, the importance of communities and their beliefs make it necessary to add the social dimension to any consideration of moral duties [27–30].

Many orientations in the training of physicians and researchers in ethical decision-making start by requesting them to examine the emotions a particular situation or state of affairs provoke. In point of fact, the philosopher Hume defined value as the power of a person or thing to evoke 'moral sentiments' related to other persons. From the initial dialogue 'within' a person's own conscience, ethical analysis proceeds to the dialogue 'between' persons and 'among' human beings. Research ethics training is already an accepted part of scientific education. In psychiatry, it acquires special features. Being a specialized profession that shares the ethos of medicine, of science and of the humanities, it adds to the problems encountered in biomedicine those related to dealing with persons whose very personhood may be in question, like those suffering of dementia and major psychoses, or are related to the influence of interpersonal factors in the application of scientific knowledge. Value-free psychiatric diagnosis may be difficult to establish. The very nature of psychotropic medication is such that its effects depend not only on chemical structure or physiological effects but also on expectations and personal interactions. Thus, problems such as placebo effects or social modulation and treatment compliance, acquire a different dimension in psychiatry than they have in general medicine.

Patient or Research Subject (Participant)?

Although intuitively attracted to think of the psychiatric profession as a research-based activity, few practitioners go over the different steps of the research process in order to achieve certainties or fundamental practices. Most of the time, they are faced with prudently contextualizing and applying knowledge generated by the social system of research using methods and under conditions not familiar to therapists. When practitioners are engaged in generating knowledge they might be tempted to rely on their role as healthcare providers and derive authority from it. This is confusing for patients who not always understand that the role of a research participant (proband or subject) is different from being a patient and, most importantly, that the role played by the professional is based on different motivations and interests. This therapeutic misunderstanding or misconception arises from different perceptions [31]. The researcher-clinician may be eager to recruit patients for a study and, in the course of such attempt, may promise unrealistic results. Or there may be a misrepresentation of what a phase I clinical trial entails. On the side of the patient ('sick people'), there may be unwarranted expectations about a procedure not yet thoroughly tested. Patients in the role of subjects cannot expect the same treatment as when in the role of 'sick persons' or patients proper. Sometimes the clinician conducting a clinical trial inadvertently 'advertises' his activity in order to recruit patients as subjects.

Avoiding Ethical Confusions: The Know-Do Gap as a Challenge in Psychosomatics

The ethics of patient care is guided by the application of principles somewhat different than the ethics of clinical research. If it is true that non-maleficence, autonomy, justice and beneficence are universal, solidarity with a fellow human being who suffers is an outstanding value in the practice of psychiatry as in other professions dealing with persons. The patient-clinician relationship is different from the subject-investigator one. The latter is incorporated into a system of interests which also includes sponsors, money-giving institutions, industrial interests, academic pressures, and love for truth. In psychiatry, as in other research-based professions, the translation of knowledge into practice faces the so-called know-do gap. This affects particularly those societies and groups that receive the results of scientific research but are unable to profit from them due to financial or procedural constraints. Practitioners in the developing countries or whose clientele has no access to adequate mental health coverage, face the situation that they know what to do or what drug to use but cannot make a sensible indication due to lack of resources [33]. The know-do gap presents an ethical dilemma in the field of public health and affects even affluent societies with minorities unable to have access to the benefits of scientific research. This should lead to reconsider research agendas in the light of their applicability to real-life situations without losing the criteria and perspectives of sound science.

As a useful guide to evaluate ethics at the research-practice interface, we use a three-dimensional approach: every project that leads to an innovation should be assessed considering whether it is good, appropriate and just. Good means well done, according to 'state-of-the-art' requirement, appropriate means right according to ethical principles, and just alludes to its generalizability as a public good. Investigators should become aware of the complexities of the challenges beyond data collection and publication. The ethics of research in psychiatry is also the ethics of the prudent application of knowledge [34]

Conclusion and Future Perspectives

Bioethics has established itself as an indispensable ancillary discourse in psychiatric practice and research. Although it has not yet challenged professional power in a very direct form, we can anticipate that it will continue making expert claims susceptible to public inquiry and amenable to open discussion. Medicine will be challenged and changed as a profession based on research, since acquisition, dissemination, and use of knowledge will be subject to public scrutiny. The good side of the coin is that it will become more accessible. The problems might be a restriction on the freedom to pursue research, and the establishment of a more direct relationship with political or economic power. The medical-industrial complex will retain power and accommodate its arguments to the ethical climate of a society in which knowledge will become a public good and its stakeholders will achieve a greater equality of access to it and its benefits. The know-do gap is expected to diminish but not in a form that makes the benefits of science equally relevant or accessible to the totality of the world population. Abstract philosophical speculation will be enriched by a more synthetic view, emphasizing the empirical aspects and conditions under which psychiatric knowledge, as a justified, true belief, is harmonized with moral considerations in the context of cultural traditions [35]. From a practical point of view, the question will remain: '*who* and in *what forms* can authorize research considering autonomy, justice, and other relevant principles' [36]. The psychosomatic approach and the problem of diagnosis will continue to be at the center of a humane care based on research and science [37, 38], irrespective of the many opinions and philosophical speculations about what mind, body, soul and thought may be as objects of study or belief.

References

1 Council for International Organizations of Medical Sciences: International Ethical Guidelines for Biomedical Research Involving Human Subjects. Geneva, CIOMS, 2002.

2 Lolas F: The axiological dimension in psychiatric diagnosis. Acta Bioethica 2009;15:148–150.

3 Sadock BJ, Sadock VA, Ruiz P (eds): Kaplan & Sadock's Comprehensive Textbook of Psychiatry. Philadelphia, Lippincott, Williams & Wilkins, 2009.

4 Lolas F: Psychiatry: medical specialty or specialized profession? World Psychiatry 2010;9:34–35.

5 Lolas F: Bioethics and psychiatry: a challenging future. World Psychiatry 2002;1:127–128.

6 Cardozo C, Mrad de Osorio A, Martínez C, Rodríguez E, Lolas F (eds): The Animal as Experimental Subject. Technical and Ethical Issues (in Spanish). Santiago, Centro Interdisciplinario de Estudios en Bioética, Universidad de Chile, 2007.

7 Lolas F: Ethics in psychiatry: a framework. World Psychiatry 2006;5:185–187.

8 Honderich T (ed): The Oxford Companion to Philosophy. Oxford, Oxford University Press, 2005.

9 Jonsen AR, Veatch RM, Walters LR (eds): Source Book in Bioethics. A Documentary History. Washington, Georgetown University Press, 1998.

10 Reich WT (ed): Encyclopedia of Bioethics. New York, Macmillan Library Reference, 1995.

11 Lolas F: Bioethics. Moral Dialogue in the Life Sciences. Santiago, Editorial Universitaria, 1999.

12 Weindling PJ: Nazi Medicine and the Nuremberg Trials: From Medical War Crimes to Informed Consent. London, Palgrave, 2004.

13 Eckart W: Human experimentation and the rights of subjects in xxth Century medicine (German); in: Psychiatrische Forschung und NS 'Euthanasie'. Heidelberg, Wunderhorn, 2001, pp 247–263.

14 Emanuel EJ, Grady C, Crouch RA, Lie RK, Miller FG, Wendler D: The Oxford Textbook of Clinical Research Ethics. Oxford, Oxford University Press, 2008.

15 Beauchamp TL, Childress JF: Principles of Biomedical Ethics, ed 5. New York, Oxford University Press, 2001.

16 Lolas F: On moral constructivism: the need for an empirical axiography (in Spanish). Acta Bioethica 2009;6:219–229.

17 Widdershoven G, Abma T, Molewijk B: Empirical ethics as dialogical practice. Bioethics 2009;23:236–248.

18 Illes J, Bird SJ: Neuroethics: a modern context for ethics in neuroscience. Trends Neurosci 2006;29:511–517.

19 Moreno JD: Neuroethics: an agenda for neuroscience and society. Nat Rev Neurosci 2003;4:149–153.

20 Farah M: Neuroethics: the practical and the philosophical. Trends Cogn Sci 2005;9:34–40.

21 Cheung EH: A new ethics of psychiatry: neuroethics, neuroscience, and technology. J Psychiatr Practice 2009;15:391–401.

22 Levy N, Clarke S: Neuroethics and psychiatry. Curr Opin Psychiatry 2008;21:568–571.

23 United Nations Educational and Scientific Organization: Establishing Bioethics Committees. Paris, UNESCO, 2005.

24 Speers MA: Evaluating the effectiveness of institutional review boards; in Emanuel EJ, Grady C, Crousch RA, Lie RK, Miller FG, Wendler D (eds): The Oxford Textbook of Clinical Research Ethics. Oxford, Oxford University Press, 2008, pp 560–568.

25 Deter HC (ed): General Clinical Medicine. Medical Praxis in Dialogue as a Fundament of a New Art of Healing (in German). Göttingen, Vandenhoeck & Ruprecht, 2007.

26 Schneider PL, Bramstedt KA: When psychiatry and bioethics disagree about patient decision making capacity (DMC). J Med Ethics 2006;32:90–93.

27 Holm S, Harris J: The standard of care in multinational research; in Emanuel EJ, Grady C, Crousch RA, Lie RK, Miller FG, Wendler D (eds): The Oxford Textbook of Clinical Research Ethics. Oxford, Oxford University Press, 2008, pp 729–736.

28 London AJ: Responsiveness to host community health needs; in Emanuel EJ, Grady C, Crousch RA, Lie RK, Miller FG, Wendler D (eds): The Oxford Textbook of Clinical Research Ethics. Oxford, Oxford University Press, 2008, pp 737–744

29 Lolas F: Psychiatry and human rights in Latin America: ethical dilemmas and the future. Internat Rev Psychiatr 2010;22:325–329.

30 Nuffield Council on Bioethics: The Ethics of Research Related to Healthcare in Developing Countries. London, Nuffield Council, 2002.

31 Appelbaum PS, Lidz CW: The therapeutic misconception; in Emanuel EJ, Grady C, Crousch RA, Lie RK, Miller FG, Wendler D (eds): The Oxford Textbook of Clinical Research Ethics. Oxford, Oxford University Press, 2008, pp 633–644.

32 Lolas F: Intercultural communication and informed consent; in Levine RJ, Gorovitz S, Gallagher S (eds): Biomedical Research Ethics: Updating International Guidelines. A Consultation. Geneva, Council for International Organizations of Medical Sciences (CIOMS), 2000, pp 135–140.

33 Lolas F, Drumond JF: Fundaments of a Bioethical Anthropology. The Good, the Appropriate and the Just (in Portuguese). Sao Paulo, Edicoes Loyola, 2007.

34 Chen DT: Curricular approaches to research ethics training for psychiatric investigators. Psychopharmacology 2003;171:112–119.

35 Carter MA: A synthetic approach to bioethical inquiry. Theor Med Bioethics 2000;21:217–234.

36 Chong SA, Huxtable R, Campbell A: Authorizing psychiatric research: principles, practices and problems. Bioethics 2011;25:27–36.

37 Lolas F: The psychosomatic approach and the problem of diagnosis. Soc Sci Med (Oxford) 1985;21:1355–1361.

38 Lolas F: Medical praxis: an interface between ethics, politics, and technology. Soc Sci Med (Oxford) 1994;39:1–5.

Fernando Lolas, MD
Department of Psychiatry, University Hospital
Interdisciplinary Center for Bioethics, University of Chile
Diagonal Paraguay 265 – Office 806, Santiago (Chile)
E-Mail flolas@u.uchile.cl

Alarcón RD (ed): Cultural Psychiatry.
Adv Psychosom Med. Basel, Karger, 2013, vol 33, pp 123–129 (DOI: 10.1159/000349900)

Epilogue

Renato D. Alarcón

Mayo Clinic College of Medicine, Rochester, Minn., USA

This volume has attempted to show a panoramic view of concepts, goals, practice and research of contemporary cultural psychiatry across the world and in its increasingly broader points of contact with other medical disciplines. As evidence of its all-encompassing perspectives, a primary notion is that of a growing visibility of cultural psychiatry taking place now, together with well-documented advances in the many fields of neurosciences. The globalization phenomena determined by migrations of all kinds and causes, and technological progress increasing (and complicating) communication networks are two of the main factors in this development: medicine as responsible for the health of world populations, and psychiatry as essential repository of medical knowledge and medical humanism cannot, therefore, ignore the challenging impact of cultural factors in the etiopathogenesis, diagnosis, treatment, outcomes and prevention of mental disorders. At the same time, research, bioethics and didactic efforts must respond to the same challenges rounding up the best and most comprehensive confrontation of disease and other plagues around the globe.

General Perspective

Cultural issues permeate all layers of medicine and psychiatry (see chapter by Alarcón). Added to the macro- and microfactors of sociocultural nature in the causality of mental disorders, biocultural connections are the subject of fascinating and promising correlational studies of biochemical, neuroimaging-based and genetic themes. The clinical presentation of many conditions is dressed up by powerful cultural characteristics that, if not well detected or understood, could lead to diagnostic or therapeutic fiascos. This, in turn, emphasizes the need to refine diagnostic practices with a full assessment of the cultural identity of the patient and his/her family, the description and explanatory models provided for each and every clinical condition, and the cultural ingredients of any therapeutic strategy. The latter must include pharmacological (enhanced by ethnic variations in the new science of pharmacogenomics) and psychotherapeutic (applicable to different modalities or schools) precisions. Last but not least, prevention in psychiatry and mental health implies education at all levels of the developmental cycle, including the enhancement of resiliency from the family nest to the social scenario.

Culture and Psychiatric Diagnosis

American psychiatry will no doubt enter into a new, possibly complicated phase of development, at least in the diagnostic field, with the use of the recently introduced fifth version of the Diagnostic and Statistical Manual of Mental Disorders (DSM-5). The cultural emphasis in DSM-5 focuses on an accurate description of the contextual elements of diagnosis and the culturally relevant material every clinician is expected to include about every patient in the characterization of each disorder. Such was the essence of discussions in a specially appointed subgroup within APA's DSM-5 Committee, presented in the chapter by Lewis-Fernández and Aggarwal. DSM-5 recommends the use of a newly developed Cultural Formulation Interview (CFI), and acknowledges the value of a comprehensive cultural assessment through a new set of 'cultural concepts of distress'. Using a dimensional approach to the clinical assessment, the subgroup ascertains a more solid diagnostic accuracy. An introductory chapter proposed to the DSM-5 Committee insisted on the clinical usefulness and the research relevance of the study of culture's influence on mental health and illness.

The CFI will enhance the notion that DSM-IV's Outline for Cultural Formulation (included in its appendix I) was the most important contribution of anthropology to clinical psychiatry and, by operationalizing it, will provide tangible methods to increase the cultural/contextual validity of psychiatric diagnosis. As part of a routine mental health evaluation, the CFI is a practical tool carefully designed to explore the patient's cultural definition of the problem, his/her cultural perceptions of cause, context and support, self-coping and help-seeking patterns. The achievement of an as clear as possible cultural identity of the patient is its main goal, and its expansion to other informants will add to the value of the data to be collected. It is clear that, beyond its clinical application, the CFI will certainly be a valuable research tool.

The newly created Glossary of Cultural Concepts of Distress puts an end to the notion of culture-bound syndromes, elaborating pragmatic definitions and examples of cultural syndromes, idioms of distress and perceived cultural causes of the clinical and behavioral occurrences. These will also have to be elaborated in the course of the clinical interview. Finally, culturally relevant material included in the descriptive text of each disorder reinforces the quality of the existing data on cultural variations, and enriches the cultural perspective of all clinicians.

International Scope of Cultural Psychiatry

The following three chapters present realities of cultural psychiatry applications and practice in five European countries. They show fascinating commonalities as well as equally intriguing differences that most probably speak out of (well!) cultural differences. The United Kingdom, a historical colonial power, focuses its cultural psychiatry practice on groups that differ in cultural heritage, particularly race, ethnicity or religion (see chapter by Bhui). Interestingly, sociology, psychology, history, health services research and public health sciences mostly applied to immigrant populations have characterized the focus and forged powerful theoretical movements or schools of thought. In recent years, there have been strong attempts at linking UK Cultural Psychiatry with world trends represented by the World Psychiatric Association (WPA), its Transcultural Psychiatry Section and the recently founded World Association of Cultural Psychiatry (WACP). Together with positive developments, concerns about social justice, resources and public health/mental health strategies emerge at the core of cultural psychiatry in its British perspective.

The main similarity between the UK and countries in continental Europe such as the Nordic Sweden and Norway and the most central Germany is their focus on mental health care access for refugees, migrants and minorities, whereas the main differences reside in their realization of having become highly culturally diverse nations. The public health-inspired financial policies, reflected in tax-funded health services and equity-based ideological principles (particularly in the Scandinavian countries) still confront needs of a culturally sensitive care in the three countries (see chapter by Bäärnhielm, Jávo and Mösko). Examples of integrated Care do exist in all of them, stimulated by facts such as Sweden and Norway's ranking among the most migration-friendly countries, or Germany's financial weight and its attached political responsibilities. Of interest, research on cultural issues in mental health care is prominent in these three countries and educational and training efforts have gained attention and prominence on the road to the materialization of truly pluralistic societies, the coexistence and coevolution of diverse human traditions, one of the most priced goals of cultural psychiatry.

The historical trajectory of French Psychiatry is universally recognized as iconic in the development of world psychiatry. After a brief review of such history and of the contributions of notable social scientists, the chapter by Westermeyer describes France's struggles for cultural homogeneity through efforts in religion, language and education led by a unique conception of geographically centralized political power. It also points out the re-emergence of cultural pride on the side of French original ethnic groups, and the realities of massive immigration from close and distant countries (particularly North Africa and the Middle East) as factors of defying strength against the homogenizing forces. The intellectual thirst of French psychiatrists and mental health professionals, plus the increasing links with other European countries and North American psychiatry have resulted in cogent contributions to the clinical and cultural angles of psychopathology. This reciprocal intellectual and scholarly nourishment (extended even to the fields of psychiatry and philosophy) can be considered a stamp unique to the image of French cultural psychiatry.

Somatization and Culture: A Critical Juncture

A volume devoted to Cultural Psychiatry and made possible by the sponsorship of a publication like *Advances in Psychosomatic Medicine*, must have as one of its nuclear contents, the examination of the clinical phenomena of somatization. The chapter by Bagayogo, Interian and Escobar does it, using once again DSM-based guidelines for the symptomatological enumerations, and historical reviews of a concept that embraces vivid clinical descriptions and still keeps an enigmatic etiology while being profusely covered and expressed by a variety of cultural connotations. The most important features in this review are the many ethnic variations of somatic symptoms and their presence both as an autonomous or semi-autonomous clinical entity, and an important component of specific clinical conditions such as depression. That some ethnic groups such as Latinos tend to report more somatic symptoms (pain, being one of the most pervasive) than Caucasian patients is, in itself, a critical warning for clinicians. Their impact on syndromic configurations, illness models and stigma-induced individual and group effects (all, cultural occurrences) is both a dramatic clinical reality and a challenging research option.

Culture and Psychiatric Treatments: Psychotherapy and Ethnopsychopharmacology

As we enter into the field of psychiatric treatment vis-à-vis culture, psychotherapy is perhaps its most subtle and most powerful aspect. In this topic, every self-respectful clinician must know the contribution of Jerome D. Frank, matter of the study of demoralization in the chapter by de Figueiredo and Gostoli. The review of the theoretical background, the methodological challenges facing research, and the clinical applications of these concepts are all areas that Frank intuited and developed rather wisely. As one of several 'common ingredients' in the path of every psychotherapy and without necessarily being clinically measurable, Demoralization is engaged with other classical concepts by stellar academic and research figures (Leighton, Kluckhorn, Jaspers) to shape up the 'assumptive world' patients bring to providers in their search for help.

In spite of these rich theoretical bases, there are only a few comparative research studies across nations and cultures. Demoralization case identification is a crucial step before attempting psychotherapy and, even more so, before planning or conducting psychotherapy. The separation between and the relief of distress vs. subjective incompetence is achieved through attempts to prevent them, to increase social support and/or raise the patient's self-esteem. Culturally inspired psychotherapies, both Western and non-Western, elicit the catalytic effects of the therapist's image, are enhanced by the healing setting, and are guided by rationales that generate a ritual or procedure. Even psychoanalytic terms such as transference and countertransference have a cultural context; scientific research may be viewed as intrusive in the quasi-religious setting of traditional healing, reason for which methodological adaptability that, for instance, may foster culturally mediated learning and even the formation of teams of lay heath counselors and respected native healers may constitute appropriate heuristic resources.

The other side of the culture-therapy connection is represented by the emerging fields of ethnopsychopharmacology and pharmacogenomics (see chapter by Silva). Natural sciences' information and knowledge, herbal therapies in different aboriginal regions and populations of the world, and astute clinical observations regarding differences in response to pharmacological agents and, specifically, to psychotropic drugs by patients from different ethnicities have coalesced to constitute these two areas of practice and research. Ethnopsychopharmacology recognizes variance in the frequency of genetic polymorphisms across populations, taking into consideration the numerous exogenous factors that impact or alter pharmacological efficacy; pharmacogenomics, in turn, studies how genetic variations influence response to medications; specifically, how families of enzymes codified by genes (grouped in individual genotypes), metabolize pharmacological agents and, through the delineation of specific dosages, engender clinical responses (or phenotypes). There are ethnic variations in this response typology but nobody can say yet to what extent cultural factors (also called 'exogenous' or 'nonbiological') affect this response. Once again, research on these topics is an open and promising field.

Research in Cultural Psychiatry: Present and Future

Research is, therefore, the area that entails both the largest set of questions and the biggest number of answers to all the above enigmas. The chapter by Kirmayer and Ban starts by affirming that a 'global monoculture' is not a phenomenon about to happen any time soon. The interplay between larger cultural blocs and a great diversity of smaller cultures groups maintained through social networks and electronic media will remain as a link between communities despite distance and dispersion. To this, we must add the sometimes difficult-to-change (for different reasons) cultural make-up of health (medicine, specifically) and other professions dealing with cultural issues. Thus, methodological strategies in general cross-cultural research represent a significant first challenge. Constructs, the re-description (and subsequent reification) of human experiences through the use of several different professional languages ('looping effects') require clinical research methods but also those from history and social science.

Emerging and enduring issues in cultural psychiatry research include cultural phenomenology and the intimate nature of psychiatric disorders, the interrelationship between cognition and emotion, cultural construction of self and personhood, cultural concepts of mental disorder, and global mental health, stigma and mental health literacy. To these, we may add ecosocial models of mental illness and wellness, and the more pragmatic assessment of cultural competence, safety and efficacy. The future of cultural psychiatry, to be paved by research work, must challenge prevalent forms of reductionism and essentialism, and postulate critical neuroscience (at the intersection of anthropology, sociology, history and philosophy of science and neuroscience) as the pathway towards how biological theories in psychiatry are rooted in cultural assumptions.

Bioethical Dimensions of Cultural Psychiatry

Psychosomatics is a research-based technical discipline whose social power may ultimately depend on how scientific knowledge is obtained and applied in practice, considering cultural contexts. Such is the preamble of the chapter by Lolas dealing with bioethical dimensions of cultural psychiatry (and psychosomatics). The bioethical discourse is based on principles that are more inclusive than professional ethics and philosophical reflections: a distinction must therefore be established between bioethics, neuroethics and applied ethics. In research, rule-guided behavior (the fundamental basis of a decision) should not be confused with norm-justifiable acts of conduct. Psychiatrists aspiring to conduct research (even more, cultural research) must do more than prudently contextualizing research-based knowledge, and recognize from the start that a patient is not necessarily the same as a research subject or participant. The 'know-do' gap can be alleviated, besides thoughtful methodological and bioethical training, by principles that grade goodness, appropriateness and justness of the research project placed at the center of a truly humane care.

Teaching of Cultural Psychiatry

All of the above considerations cannot be realized without systematic and appropriate educational/didactic efforts. Medical students, residents and fellows should address their training on the basis of skills (complementing knowledge and attitudes) that include genuine cultural competence, the practical understanding of culture as an essential component of psychiatric theory and practice. Comprehensiveness, consistency and creativity are three essential ingredients of this pursuit. Comprehensiveness entails totality which does not mean neglect of the individuality of patients but the harmonious integration of methods and tools. Consistency implies certitude of goals, thoroughness of didactic strategies and commitment to keep requirements, schedules, effectiveness and efficiency of tools. Creativity reflects and assures adaptability, flexibility, visionary but also practical use of existing means and resources that can assist in the achievement of the primary goals of the educational program.

The general goals of teaching of core cultural competencies include the conduction of a well-organized clinical interview, professionalism, empathy and genuine human understanding of the patient and his/her family, the achievement of a meaningful initial diagnosis, the setting up of comprehensive tests aimed at further diagnostic precision, familiarization with institutional rules of clinical documentation, initiation and conduction of appropriately comprehensive treatment plans, as well as establishment of adequate follow-up procedures. More specific cultural components have to do with exhaustive exploration of cultural variables, the use of the CFI in search of the patient's cultural identity, recognition of racial/ethnic, social and cultural similarities and differences, elements of a possible migration history, information about family history, structural hierarchies, coping mechanisms, etc., identification of cultural risk and protective factors, cultural aspects of the primary psychopathologies (i.e. impact on severity), cultural correlates of psychometric and other tests, inclusion of adequate cultural documentation, pharmacological and pharmacogenomics clarifications, fostering of truly multidisciplinary care with a multidisciplinary team-based approach, and recognition of the sociocultural implications of the case in the context of public mental health policies and procedures.

Additional didactic tools, beyond the actual and decisive patient contact under good supervision, include readings and lectures, problem-based, case-based, patient- and trainee-centered activities, journal clubs, experiential groups, journaling by the trainees, and provision of adequate bibliographic support. The assessment of performance must be reliable, valid and practical. It will explore not only about degree of knowledge but whether the objectives for the educational experience were reached, areas in need of new acquisitions or improvement, provision of formative and summative feedback to the students, residents or fellows. Curricular design and appropriate use of electronic equipment are also indispensable parameters.

It can be said that cultural competence is a substantial component of any psychiatric practice; however, the scope of this statement is much broader when talking about knowledge, attitudes and skills in cultural psychiatry proper. Even though there are not too many cultural psychiatry training programs (i.e. fellowships), or the schedule of cultural psychiatry courses in residents' or medical students' didactic programs is scarce, basic literature sources, textbooks, articles and essays are part of the rich bibliography of all the chapters in this volume. We invite the readers to look through these pages with the interest and devotion of professionals and/or trainees deeply imbued of the genuinely human and humanistic tradition of the mental health field.

Prof. Renato D. Alarcón, MD, MPH
Emeritus Professor of Psychiatry
Mayo Clinic College of Medicine, 200 First St. S.W.
Rochester, MN 55905 (USA)
E-Mail alarcon.renato@mayo.edu

Author Index

Subject Index